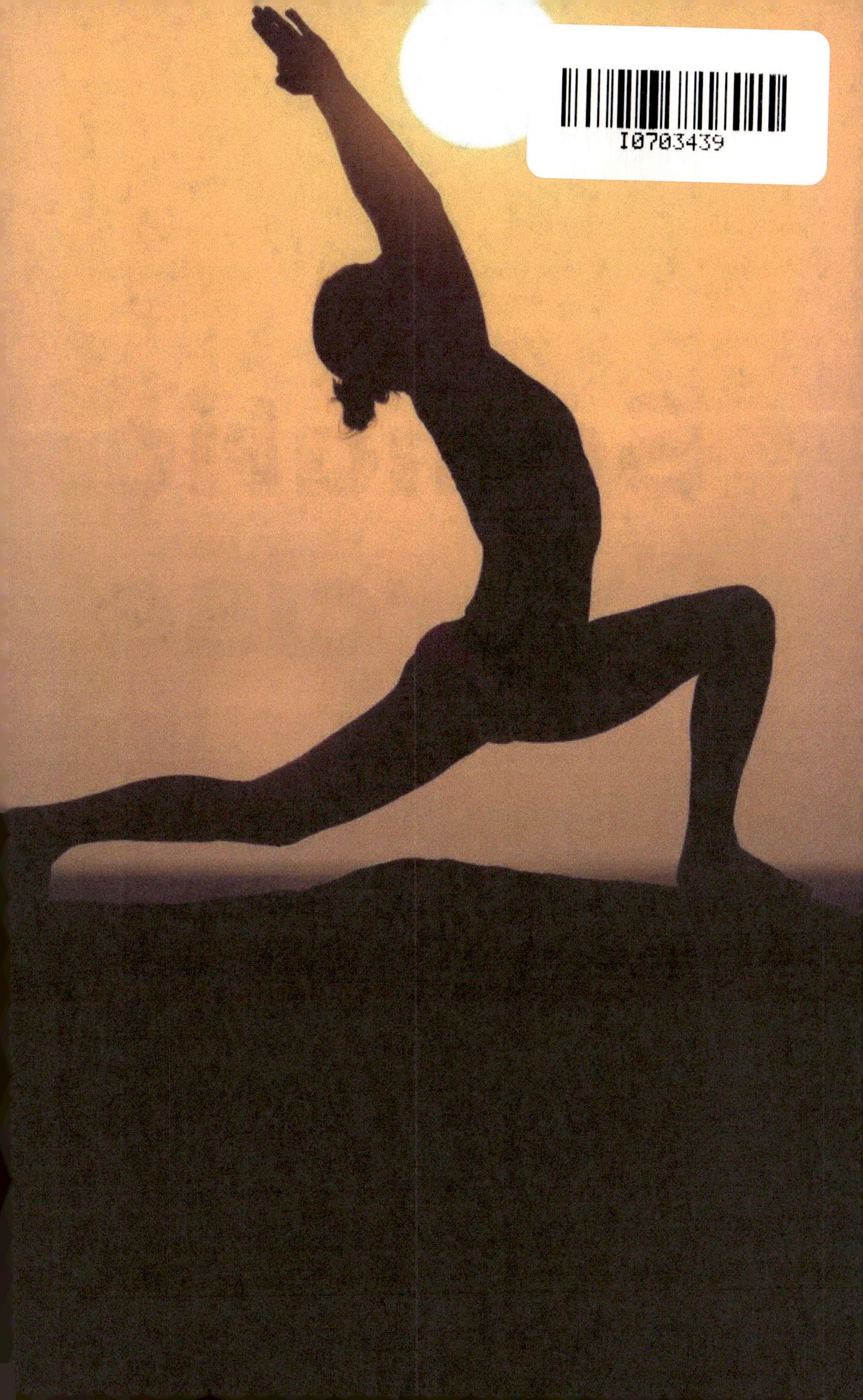
I0703439

Somatic Exercise

Comprehensive Mind-Body Practices for

Holistic Health and Wellness

Author

Beth James

Copyright © 2024 by Beth James

All rights reserved. No part of this book may be reproduced, distributed, or transmitted in any form or by any means, including photocopying, recording, or other electronic or mechanical methods, without the prior written permission of the publisher, except in the case of brief quotations embodied in critical reviews and certain other non-commercial uses permitted by copyright law.

Disclaimer:

This book is intended to provide helpful and informative material on the subjects addressed. It is not intended to replace medical advice, nor is it intended to diagnose, treat, cure, or prevent any medical condition. The author and publisher are not responsible for any adverse effects or consequences resulting from the use of any suggestions or exercises described within this book. Always consult a healthcare professional before beginning any new exercise program.

DEDICATION

To all those who relentlessly pursue physical and mental well-being, and to those who have discovered joy, strength, and healing through somatic exercises. This book is for the seekers, the healers, and the dreamers who believe in the transformative power of mindful movement. May you continue to find inspiration and renewal on your journey to body awareness and healing.

"The body never lies."
— Martha Graham

Table of Contents

FOREWORD

In "Somatic Exercises: Comprehensive Mind-Body Practices for Holistic Health and Wellness," discover the profound connection between body and mind. This book delves into somatic practices pioneered by Elsa Gindler, Moshe Feldenkrais, and Thomas Hanna, offering a rich blend of history, science, and practical application. Through mindful movements, reprogram your brain, enhance physical capabilities, and achieve emotional resilience. Whether you're a beginner or advanced practitioner, detailed routines and visual aids guide you toward stress relief, pain management, and overall well-being. Embrace this holistic approach to health, fostering deeper self-awareness and transformation. Welcome to a journey of discovery and harmony, where the path to holistic wellness begins.

PREFACE

Welcome to "Somatic Exercises: Comprehensive Mind-Body Practices for Holistic Health and Wellness." This book is born from years of experience and aims to guide you on a transformative journey, bridging body and mind for holistic health. Inspired by pioneers Elsa Gindler, Moshe Feldenkrais, and Thomas Hanna, this guide offers practical routines and modifications for all levels. Discover how somatic exercises relieve pain, reduce stress, and foster emotional healing. Each chapter provides detailed instructions, visual aids, and tips for integrating practices into daily life. Embrace this journey with an open mind, exploring your body's capabilities and achieving greater harmony and well-being. Welcome to your path to holistic wellness.

CHAPTER 1: INTRODUCTION TO SOMATIC EXERCISES

Definition and History of Somatic Exercises

Somatic exercises are a holistic means of maintaining health concerning the experience taking place within one's own body. The word "somatic" is derived from the Greek word "soma," which means "living body." Somatic exercises create awareness and foster well-being in and around the body, enable better movement patterns, and promote overall health by being a bridge to connect the body and mind.

Somatic exercises were first pioneered in the early 20th century by such pioneers as Elsa Gindler, Moshe Feldenkrais, and Thomas Hanna. Elsa Gindler was a German educator who developed movement-based therapies for greater awareness of bodily sensations. The Feldenkrais Method is a method developed by an Israeli physicist and engineer, Moshe Feldenkrais, to improve human functioning and reduce pain through the use of gentle movements and directed attention. Thomas Hanna, an American philosopher and movement educator, coined the term "somatics" and created Hanna Somatic Education for those plagued with chronic tension and disorders of movement.

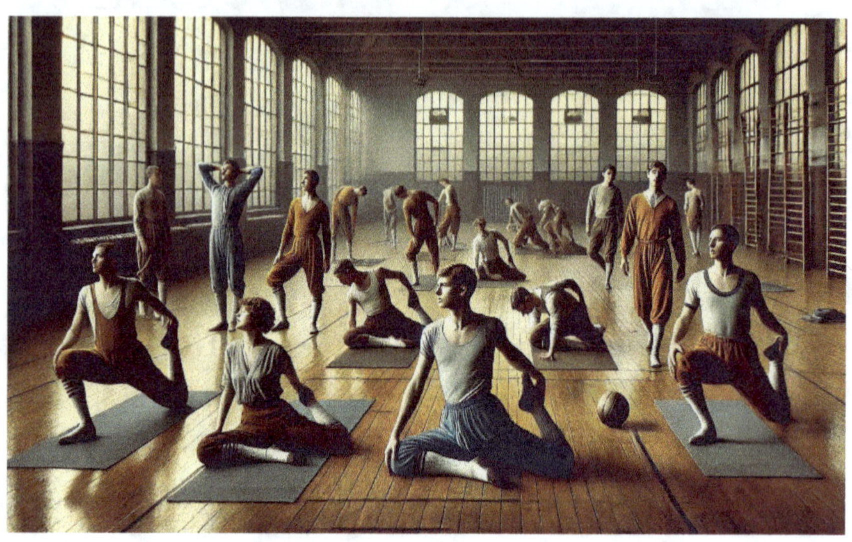

These fundamental methods have been developed and incorporated over decades with other practices, such as yoga, Pilates, mindfulness meditation, and somatic exercises, which have formed a wide body of practice. These methods could be further specialized for a number of needs and preferences.

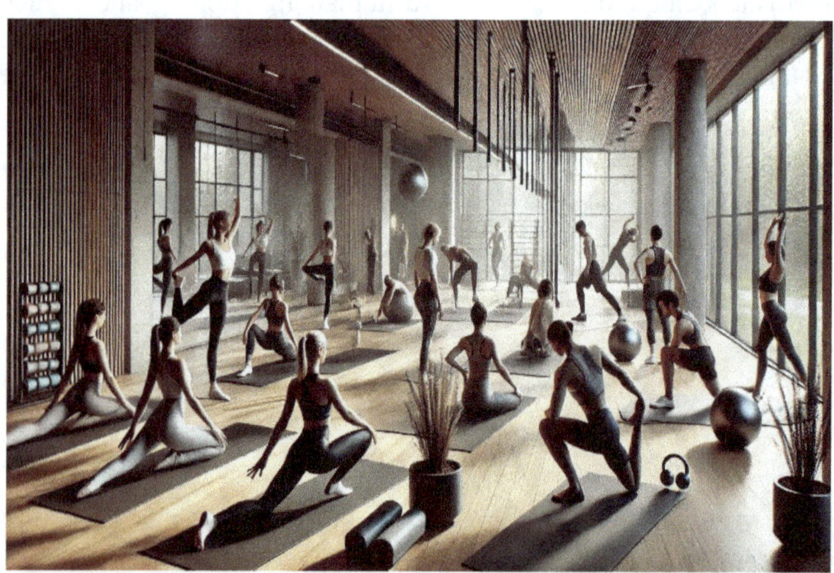

The Science and Benefits of Somatic Exercises

Somatic exercises are based on neuroplasticity, the science of the brain's ability to reorganize itself by forming new neural connections throughout life. The importance of this concept is that it explains how repetitive mindful movements do, in fact, go on to change the brain and, hence, improve how your body functions.

In somatic exercises, we deliberately pay attention to different body parts and the movements they make. Such an act reprograms the brain through the increase in proprioception—the sense of body position—and kinaesthesia—the sense of body movement. Better coordination, balance, and performance are then enhancement benefits for improved proprioception and kinaesthesia.

Benefits of somatic exercise

1. **Pain Relief**: This is affected as somatic exercises assist in the identification and then the release of chronic muscle tension. This reduces the pain or discomfort, especially for those experiencing pain in the back, neck, and joints.

2. Enhance Flexibility and Mobility: Somatic exercises provide movements that are smooth and natural, which enhance flexibility and mobility. It can be particularly helpful in dealing with older adults and people who are undergoing rehabilitation.

3. Stress Reduction: Somatic exercises are mindful and encourage relaxation, hence reducing stress. The person performing this exercise lives in the present moment and in his or her body; it is a way to attain calmness and clarity of mind.

4. Enhanced Body Awareness: Regular practice of somatic exercises will increase the awareness of one's body so an individual can identify and correct poor postures and movement habits. This will manifest in him or her moving more economically and gracefully.

5. Emotional Healing: Somatic exercises can also aid with emotional healing. The body is a reservoir of great stress and trauma, so releasing the physical tension may make one realize the emotional release and healing.

6. Better General Health: Regular somatic exercise can enhance general health through better Circulation, immune system functioning, and sleep patterns.

In summary, somatic exercises offer a comprehensive approach to physical and emotional well-being. By understanding their history, principles, and benefits, individuals can embark on a journey to greater body awareness and healing, ultimately leading to a more balanced and fulfilling life.

Why Somatic Exercises

Personal Stories and Success Stories

What I have been privy to as a somatic coach goes far beyond what one might consider a dry, theoretical wish list of qualities and attributes which one might aspire to acquire. One such story is that of a 45-year-old mother of two by the name of Sarah, who had gone through a number of treatments due to the chronic back pain she was suffering from. She had tried several remedies, from physical therapy to medication, with little success.

Sarah was very skeptical when I first started her on Somatic

Exercises, but she opened her mind to it. We worked with gentle movement and focused attention on identifying the tensions and increased awareness of the body. Very slowly, Sarah began to pick up on subtle cues: her pain was starting to decrease, her posture was getting better, and she felt more connected to her body. The transformation of Sarah was more than skin deep: she also had emotional relief, wherein she felt less stress and was better able to be in the moment.

Another inspiring story is that of James, an athlete who had retired and lived a very active life but had to go through the pain of getting up with stiffness and having limited mobility after those activities. He was frustrated since he could not move freely like before to do the kind of activities he loved.

Thanks to somatic exercises, James could listen to his body and move normally. His flexibility returned, pain diminished, and the sports fire within him was kindled again. This is just the way somatic exercises bring vitality and joy in life back, even after long wear and tear on the body of a person.

These are but a few stories that show what somatic exercises can be capable of in transforming and changing the lives of individuals, addressing matters of both physical and emotional health.

Developing Body Awareness and Mindfulness

Body awareness and mindfulness are really the foundation for any somatic exercise, the true leverage point for bringing out all the full potential for living a balanced and healthy life.

Body Awareness:

The ability to perceive and understand sensations, movements and position in your body. It is the paying of attention to the feeling of how your body moves and feels when it is both still and moving. Some reasons why this awareness is important include:

Prevention of injury: you will avoid injuries from strain or poor techniques with increased body awareness of your limits and movements. For instance, knowing the weight that is lifted and how it is distributed in the body can avert hurting the back.

Good Posture and Alignment: Having body awareness also improves posture and alignment, reducing the likelihood of chronic pain. For example, knowing when you are slouching helps you make corrections to your body so you do not get pains in your neck and back.

Enhanced Physical Performance: Improved body awareness is also critical to athletes and performers. They can fine-tune their movements, which significantly improves their performance and decreases the possibility of injuries.

Emotional Insight: The emotional pain and trauma held by the body is released. Increased awareness of one's body can allow you to notice and release any resulting tensions, providing better emotional healing or possibly emotional fortitude.

Mindfulness:

It involves the full attention of a person directed into the moment of reality with an open and non-judgmental attitude. As applied in somatic exercise, here are the benefits of mindfulness: Reduced Stress: Mindfulness calms the mind; therefore, stress is highly reduced. When one is in the right state of mind, focusing on the present moment allows one to forget all their worries concerning the past or future and develop a certain feeling of peace and relaxation.

Concentration Improvement: Training in mindfulness would produce an increase in your capacity for better concentration. This will eventually enable a rise in productivity and performance in different areas of life.

Emotional Regulation: Mindfulness leads to the effective control of emotions, as it permits observing one's thoughts and feelings without becoming fully identified with them. In the process, this allows one to exert emotional control and achieve improvement in overall mental health.

Enhanced Quality of Life: Embracing mindfulness can lead you to remain fully present during activities and relationships that make you happy. Integrating Mindful Body Awareness: Somatic exercises thus beautifully blend body awareness with mindfulness, both key tools to holistic well-being. How your body feels and moves from mindful attention creates deeper intimacy with the self, hence leading to physical health, emotional resilience, and a general sense of well-being. You would experience a deep transformation in your life by including somatic exercises. The details of why somatic exercises are the way to begin realizing and healing oneself are vividly underscored by the stories shared, providing the underlying principles of body awareness and mindfulness, which easily show somatic exercises to be such a valuable and impactful practice.

It will be easier to understand what somatic exercises are if we first get familiar with how our nervous system and somatic pathways function. Here are some very simplified diagrams of those concepts:

Nervous System

There are two main divisions of the nervous system:

Central Nervous System (CNS): Made up of the brain and spinal cord, it interprets information and issues orders to the rest of the body.

Peripheral Nervous System (PNS): All the nerves of the body outside the CNS. These form connecting pathways from the brain and spinal cord to the remaining parts of the body.

Somatic Pathway

Somatic pathways: These are the ways that lead the sensory information from the body to the brain and motor command from the brain to the muscles. Somatic pathways include the following:

Sensory Pathways: The pathways upon which information travels from sensory receptors to the CNS.

Motor Pathways: These are the pathways through which the central nervous system sends signals down to the muscles for movement.

Charts Displaying Benefits and Statistics on Somatic Exercises

To this end, look at these graphs to illustrate the benefits and impact of bodily exercises.

Chart: Benefits of Somatic Exercise

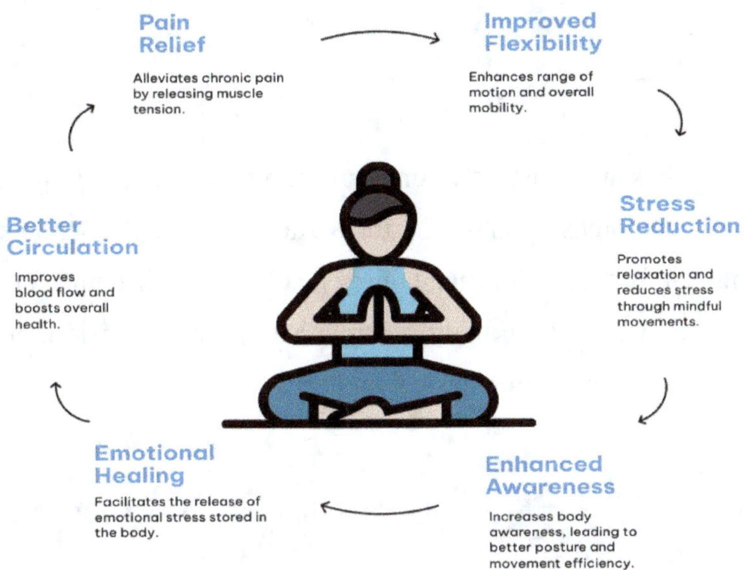

Numerical Data on the Effect of Somatic Exercises

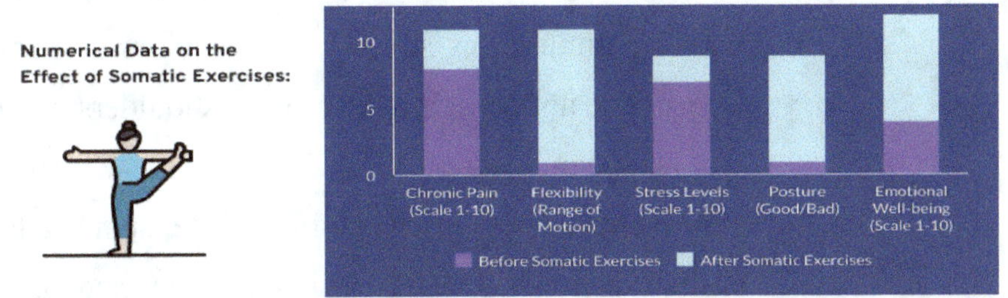

These charts and diagrams help make visual sense of how the bodily exercises actually work on the body and mind. These embeds will facilitate readers in visualizing more clearly what science and benefits are associated with somatic exercises, which makes the content both dynamic and extremely educative.

CHAPTER 2: UNDERSTANDING YOUR BODY'S SIGNALS

The Language of the Body

Our bodies are constantly communicating with us, sending signals that reflect our physical and emotional state. Learning to understand this language is crucial for maintaining health and well-being. This chapter will explore how the body communicates stress, tension, and trauma and how to recognize physical and emotional cues.

How the Body Communicates Stress, Tension, and Trauma

1. **Stress:**
   - **Muscle Tension:** One of the most common ways the body communicates stress is through muscle tension. You might notice tightness in your shoulders, neck, or jaw when you're stressed.
   - **Headaches:** Stress often manifests as tension headaches or migraines. These can be a sign that your body is under too much pressure.
   - **Digestive Issues:** The gut is highly sensitive to stress. Symptoms like stomach aches, nausea, or changes in appetite can indicate stress.
   - **Rapid Heartbeat:** An increased heart rate or palpitations can be a direct response to stress, signaling that your body is in a state of heightened alert.

2. **Tension:**

- o **Stiffness:** Chronic tension can lead to stiffness in the joints and muscles, limiting your range of motion.
- o **Aches and Pains:** Persistent aches, particularly in the back, neck, and shoulders, are common indicators of built-up tension.
- o **Fatigue:** Tension can drain your energy, leaving you feeling fatigued even after adequate rest.

3. **Trauma:**

- o **Hypervigilance:** Trauma can cause a state of hypervigilance, where the body is always on high alert, expecting danger. This can manifest as an exaggerated startle response or difficulty relaxing.
- o **Flashbacks:** The body might react to certain triggers that bring back memories of the traumatic event, leading to physical symptoms like sweating, shaking, or a racing heart.
- o **Chronic Pain:** Trauma often results in chronic pain conditions, where the body retains the physical manifestations of past injuries or stress.
- o **Emotional Numbness:** Trauma can lead to a disconnect between the body and emotions, causing feelings of numbness or detachment.

Recognizing Physical and Emotional Cues

1. **Physical Cues:**

- o **Posture:** Notice your posture throughout the day. Are you slumping forward or holding your body rigidly? Poor posture can be a sign of underlying stress or tension.

- o **Breathing Patterns:** Pay attention to your breath. Shallow, rapid breathing can indicate anxiety or stress, while deep, slow breaths usually signal relaxation.
- o **Facial Expressions:** Your face can reveal a lot about your internal state. Tightness around the eyes or mouth, furrowed brows, or clenched jaws can indicate stress or tension.
- o **Body Temperature:** Sudden changes in body temperature, like feeling hot or cold without an apparent reason, can be a response to emotional stress or anxiety.

2. **Emotional Cues:**
   - o **Mood Swings:** Frequent changes in mood can be a sign that your body is under stress. Pay attention to how your emotions fluctuate throughout the day.
   - o **Irritability:** Feeling unusually irritable or short-tempered can indicate that your body is dealing with stress or unresolved tension.
   - o **Anxiety:** Persistent feelings of anxiety or unease are strong indicators that your body is responding to stress or trauma.
   - o **Depression:** Symptoms of depression, such as feelings of hopelessness, fatigue, or a lack of interest in activities you once enjoyed, can be related to chronic stress or unresolved trauma.

Practical Steps to Enhance Body Awareness

1. **Mindful Check-ins:** Set aside a few minutes each day to do a mindful check-in with your body. Close your eyes, take a few deep breaths, and mentally scan your body from head to toe.

Notice any areas of tension, discomfort, or unusual sensations.

2. **Journaling:** Keep a journal to track your physical and emotional states. Note any patterns or recurring symptoms and reflect on possible triggers or contributing factors. This practice can help you become more attuned to your body's signals.

3. **Movement Practices:** Engage in movement practices like yoga, tai chi, or gentle stretching. These activities promote body awareness and help release tension. Pay attention to how your body feels before, during, and after these sessions.

4. **Breathwork:** Practice conscious breathing techniques to enhance your body awareness and reduce stress. Techniques like diaphragmatic breathing or alternate nostril breathing can help you connect with your body's signals and promote relaxation.

5. **Professional Guidance:** Consider working with a somatic therapist or coach who can guide you in developing greater body awareness and understanding your body's signals. Professional support can provide personalized strategies and insights to help you on your journey.

By learning to recognize and interpret the language of your body, you can take proactive steps towards better health and emotional well-being. Understanding your body's signals is the first step in addressing stress, tension, and trauma and, ultimately, achieving a more balanced and harmonious life.

Mind-Body Connection

Exploring the Relationship Between Mental and Physical Health
The mind-body connection is a fundamental concept in understanding overall health and well-being. This relationship emphasizes that our

mental state can significantly impact our physical health and vice versa. Here's a comprehensive exploration of this connection:

The Relationship Between Mental and Physical Health

1. **Stress and Physical Health:**
   - **Immune System:** Chronic Stress can weaken the immune system, making the body more susceptible to infections and illnesses.
   - **Cardiovascular Health:** Prolonged Stress increases the risk of heart disease by causing high blood pressure, elevated cholesterol levels, and increased heart rate.
   - **Digestive System:** Stress can lead to digestive problems such as irritable bowel syndrome (IBS), acid reflux, and stomach ulcers.

2. **Mental Health and Chronic Pain:**
   - **Pain Perception:** Mental health conditions like depression and anxiety can amplify the perception of pain, making chronic pain conditions more debilitating.
   - **Inflammation:** Depression is often linked to increased levels of inflammation in the body, contributing to chronic pain and other inflammatory conditions.

3. **Emotional Well-being and Physical Health:**
   - **Hormonal Balance:** Positive emotions and mental well-being can promote hormonal balance, supporting overall physical health.
   - **Physical Activity:** Good mental health encourages physical activity, which in turn enhances physical health by improving cardiovascular fitness, muscle strength, and flexibility.

4. **Psychosomatic Symptoms:**

   o **Physical Manifestations:** Psychological issues can manifest as physical symptoms, such as headaches, fatigue, and muscle tension. These symptoms are real and need to be addressed holistically.

Visual Aids

Illustrations of Common Body Signals and Their Meanings

Here are some common body signals and their possible meanings:

1. Headaches:

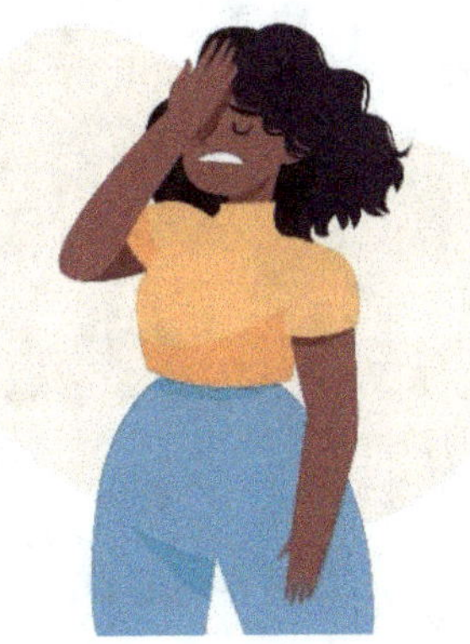

Stress: Tension headaches are often caused by stress and anxiety.

Dehydration: Lack of water intake can lead to headaches.

Poor Posture: Strain from poor posture can cause neck and head pain.

2. **Tight Shoulders:**

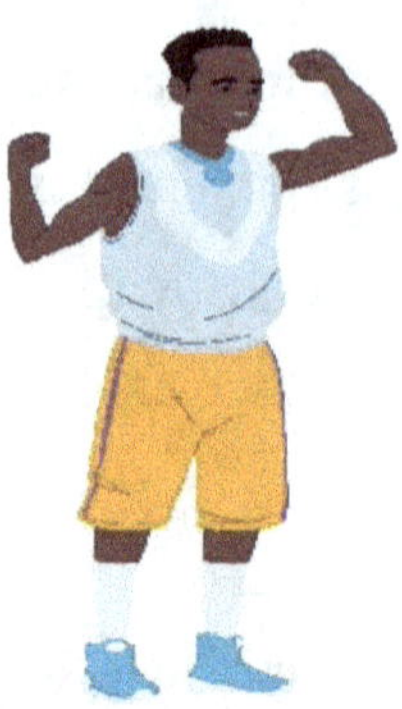

Stress: Emotional Stress often accumulates in the shoulder muscles.

Poor Ergonomics: Sitting in front of a computer with poor posture can cause shoulder tension.

3. **Stomach Issues:**

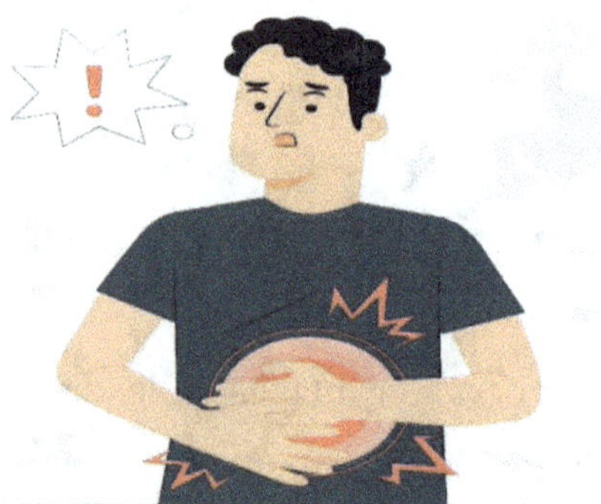

4. **Anxiety:** Anxiety can lead to digestive problems such as nausea, bloating, and stomach pain.

Diet: Poor dietary choices can cause stomach discomfort.

4. Fatigue:

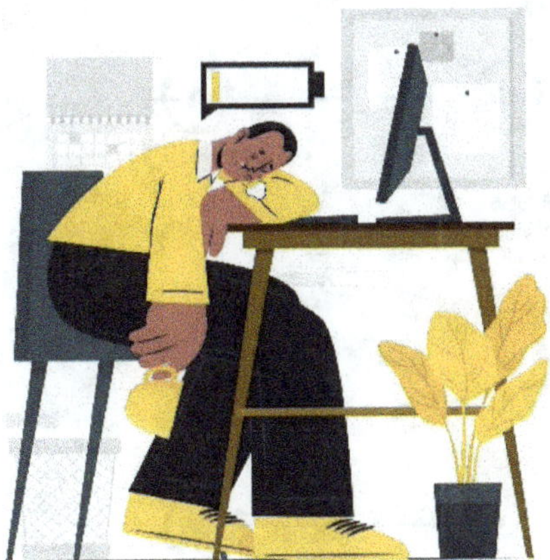

Sleep Deprivation: Lack of adequate sleep is a common cause of fatigue.

Mental Exhaustion: Mental Stress and overwork can lead to feelings of physical tiredness.

Flowcharts of Mind-Body Interaction

Below are flowcharts to illustrate the interaction between the mind and body.

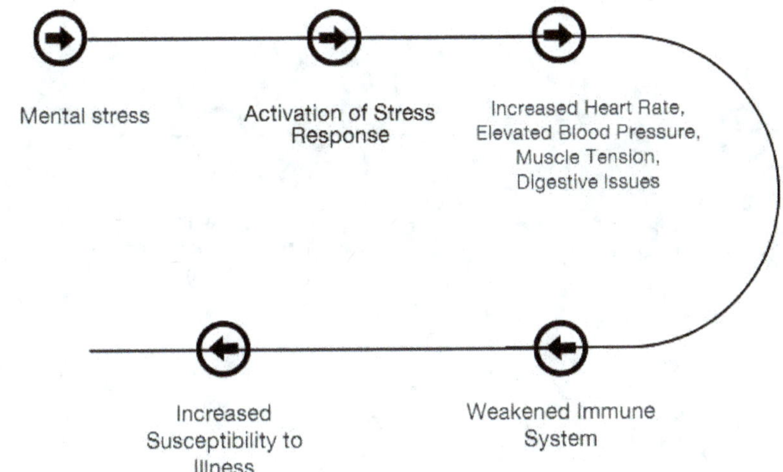

Flowchart 2: Positive Mental Health and Physical Well-being

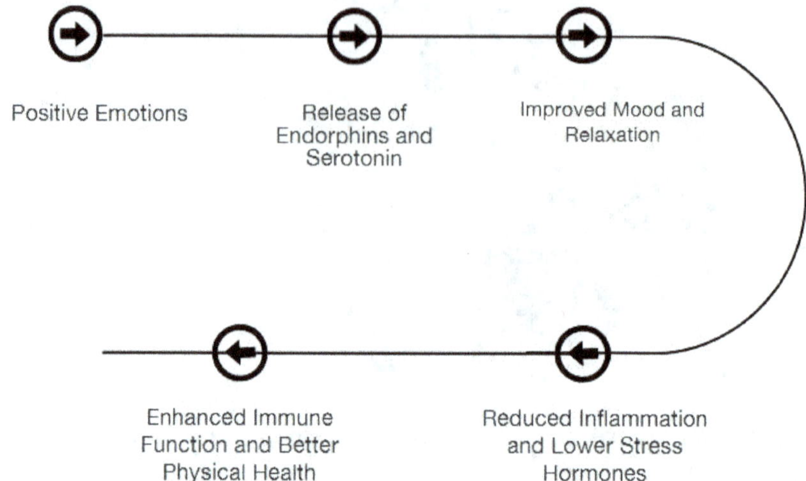

Flowchart 3: Anxiety and Its Physical Manifestations

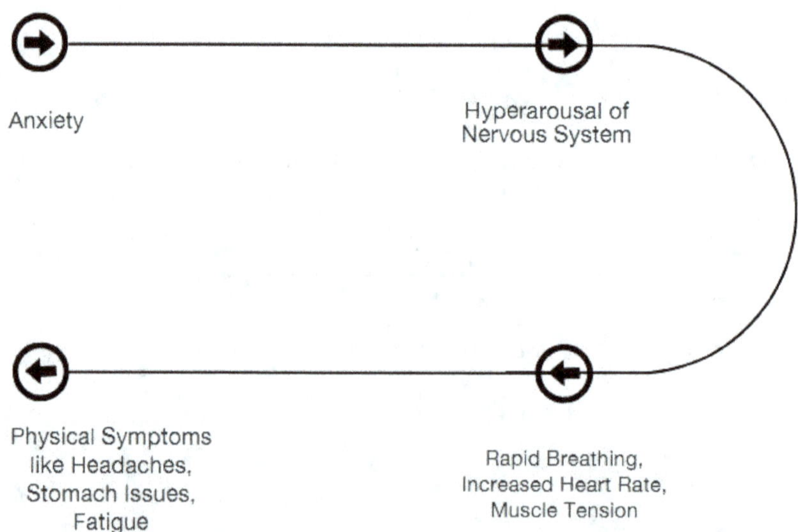

These visual aids help to clarify the complex interactions between our mental and physical health, making it easier to understand the profound impact our thoughts and emotions can have on our bodies.

By exploring the mind-body connection and using visual aids to illustrate these concepts, we can gain a deeper understanding of how to maintain holistic health. Recognizing and addressing both mental and physical aspects of well-being is essential for achieving a balanced and healthy life.

CHAPTER 3: BASIC SOMATIC EXERCISES FOR BEGINNERS

Getting Started

Preparing Your Mind and Environment for Practice

Starting a somatic exercise routine requires a mindful approach to both your mental state and your physical environment. Here's how to get started:

1. **Mind Preparation:**

- **Set Intentions:** Begin by setting clear intentions for your practice. Ask yourself what you hope to achieve—whether it's reducing stress, improving flexibility, or enhancing overall well-being. Setting intentions helps to focus your mind and provides motivation.

- **Create a Routine:** Establish a regular time for your practice. Consistency is key to developing a habit and reaping the benefits of somatic exercises. Choose a time when you are least likely to be interrupted and can fully dedicate yourself to the practice.

- **Mindfulness:** Approach your practice with a mindset of mindfulness. Be present and attentive to your body's sensations and movements. Let go of any expectations or judgments, and allow yourself to simply be in the moment.

2. **Environment Preparation:**

- **Choose a Quiet Space:** Find a quiet and comfortable space where you can practice without distractions. This could be a room in your home, a corner of your living room, or even a peaceful outdoor area.

- o **Comfortable Clothing:** Wear loose, comfortable clothing that allows for easy movement. Avoid tight or restrictive garments that can hinder your practice.

- o **Mat or Blanket:** Use a yoga mat or a soft blanket to provide cushioning for floor exercises. Ensure that the surface is non-slip and supportive.

- o **Lighting and Ambiance:** Adjust the lighting to a soft, soothing level. You might also consider playing gentle background music, or nature sounds to create a calming atmosphere.

Basic Breathing and Centering Techniques

Breathing and centering are fundamental components of somatic exercises. These techniques help to calm the mind, enhance body awareness, and prepare you for deeper practice.

1. **Diaphragmatic Breathing:**
- o **Step-by-Step Guide:**
1. Sit or lie down in a comfortable position with your back straight.
2. Place one hand on your chest and the other on your abdomen.
3. Inhale deeply through your nose, allowing your abdomen to rise as your diaphragm expands. Your chest should remain relatively still.

4. Exhale slowly through your mouth, letting your abdomen fall. Feel the air gently leaving your body.
5. Repeat for 5-10 minutes, focusing on the rise and fall of your abdomen.
- o **Benefits:** Diaphragmatic breathing reduces stress, lowers blood

pressure, and promotes relaxation. It also enhances oxygen flow, supporting overall health.

2. **4-7-8 Breathing Technique:**

o **Step-by-Step Guide:**

1. Sit comfortably with your back straight and your hands resting on your lap.

2. Close your eyes and take a deep breath in through your nose for a count of 4.

3. Hold your breath for a count of 7.

4. Exhale completely through your mouth for a count of 8, making a whooshing sound.

5. Repeat the cycle three more times for a total of four breaths.

o **Benefits:** This technique helps to reduce anxiety, improve sleep, and promote a sense of calm.

3. **Body Scan Meditation:**

o **Step-by-Step Guide:**

1. Lie down on your back with your arms at your sides, palms facing up. Close your eyes.

2. Take a few deep breaths, allowing your body to relax with each exhale.

3. Begin by focusing your attention on your toes. Notice any sensations, tension, or relaxation in this area.

4. Gradually move your focus up through your body: feet, ankles, calves, knees, thighs, hips, abdomen, chest, back, shoulders, arms, hands, neck, and finally your head.

5. Spend a few moments on each body part, observing without judgment.

6. Once you reach the top of your head, take a few more deep breaths and slowly open your eyes.

o   **Benefits:** Body scan meditation enhances body awareness, reduces stress, and promotes relaxation.

4. **Centering Technique:**

o   **Step-by-Step Guide:**

1. Stand or sit comfortably with your feet shoulder-width apart. Close your eyes.

2. Take a few deep breaths to relax your body.

3. Visualize a line of energy running from the top of your head down through the center of your body, grounding you to the earth.

4. Gently sway your body forward and backwards, side to side, finding a point of balance where you feel stable and centered.

5. Focus on this point of balance, imagining yourself as a tree with deep roots extending into the ground, providing stability and strength.

6. Take a few more deep breaths, feeling connected and centered.

o   **Benefits:** Centering helps to balance your body and mind, improve focus, and reduce feelings of stress and disorientation.

By preparing your mind and environment and practicing these basic breathing and centering techniques, you create a strong foundation for your somatic exercise journey. These practices not only enhance your body awareness but also promote a sense of calm and well-being, making it easier to engage fully with the exercises and experience their benefits.

Basic Somatic Exercises for Beginners

Simple Routines

In this section, we'll explore ten foundational somatic exercises designed to enhance body awareness, reduce tension, and promote overall well-being. Each exercise includes step-by-step instructions, tips for maintaining consistency and motivation, and visual aids for better understanding.

1. Pelvic Tilt

Step-by-Step Instructions:

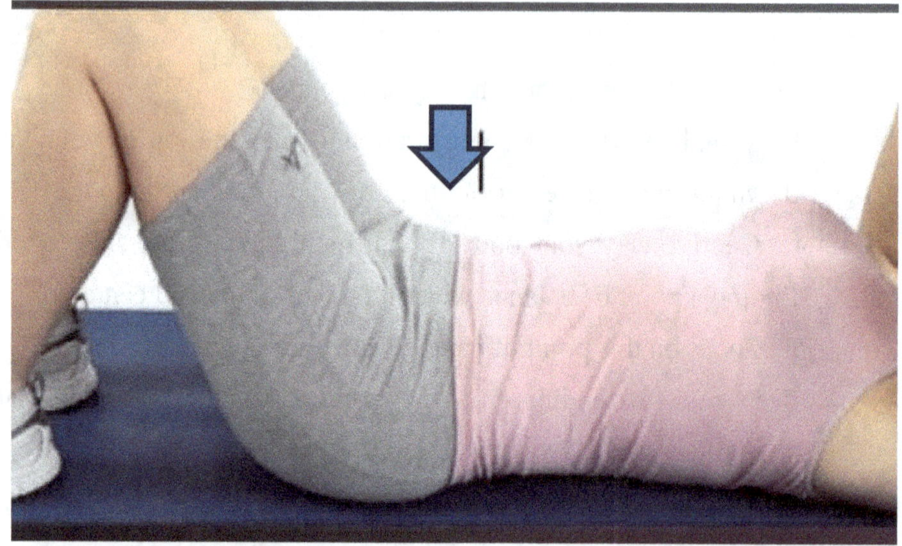

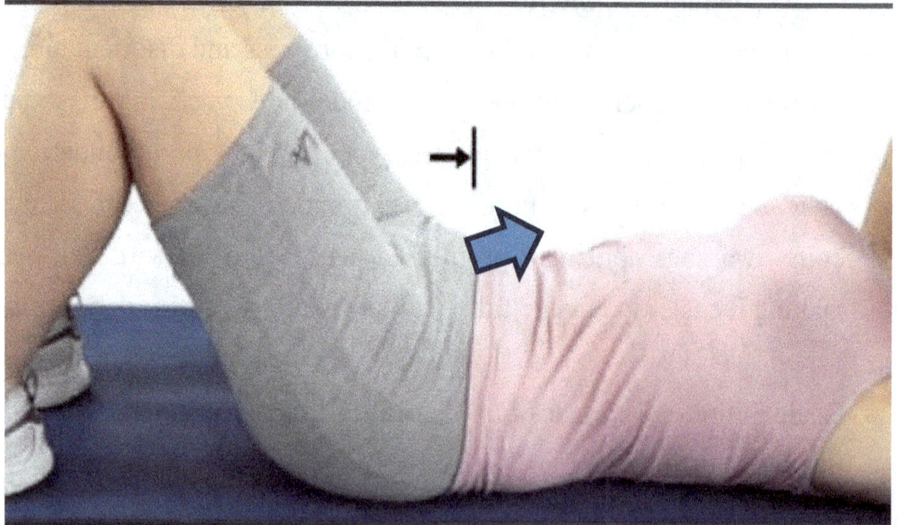

1. Lie on your back with your knees bent and feet flat on the floor, hip-width apart.

2. Place your hands on your lower abdomen.

3. Inhale deeply, then exhale and gently tilt your pelvis backwards, pressing your lower back into the floor.

4. Inhale and return to the neutral position.

5. Repeat ten times, focusing on the movement of your pelvis and lower back.

Tips:

Keep the movement slow and controlled.

Focus on the sensations in your lower back and abdomen.

Video guide: [Pelvic Tilt Video]

2. Cat-Cow Stretch

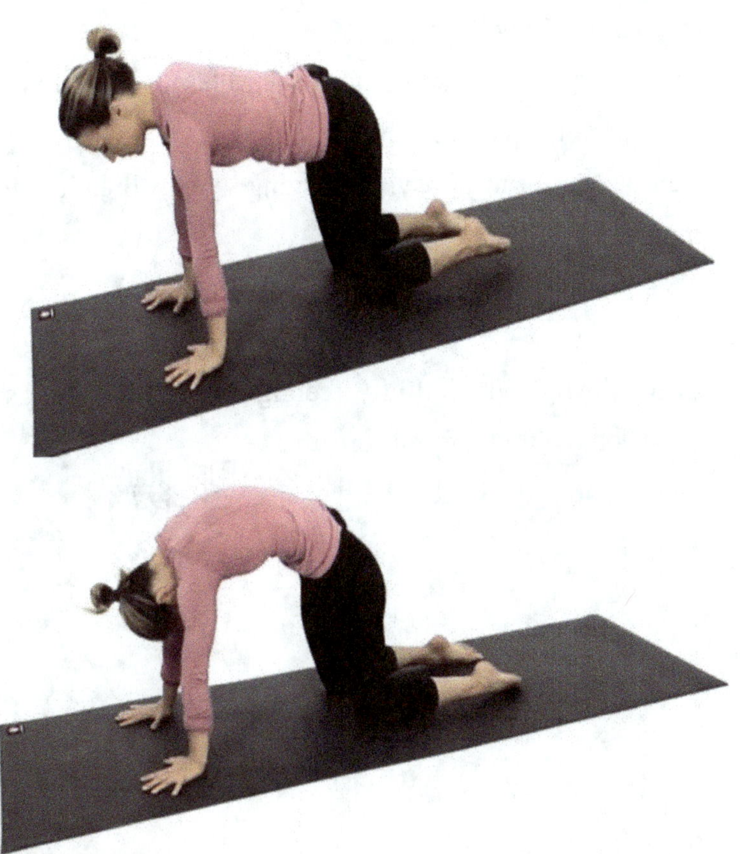

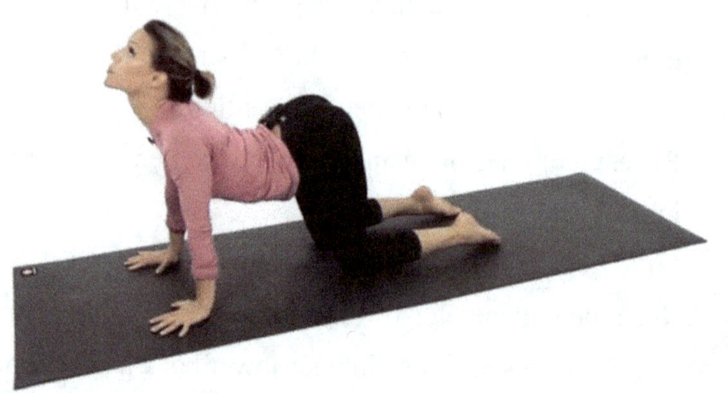

Step-by-Step Instructions:

1. Start on your hands and knees with your wrists aligned under your shoulders and knees under your hips.
2. Inhale, arch your back and lift your head and tailbone towards the ceiling (Cow Pose).
3. Exhale, round your spine, tuck your chin and draw your belly towards your spine (Cat Pose).
4. Repeat ten times, synchronizing your breath with the movements.

Tips:

Move slowly and mindfully, feeling the stretch in your spine. Focus on the flow of your breath.

Video guide: [Cat-Cow Stretch Video](#)

3. Shoulder Roll

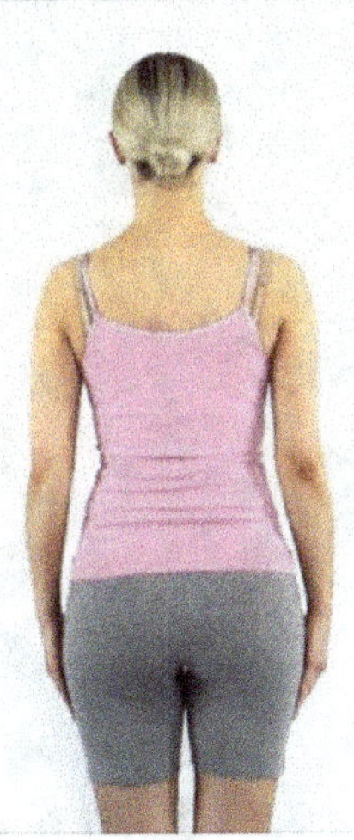

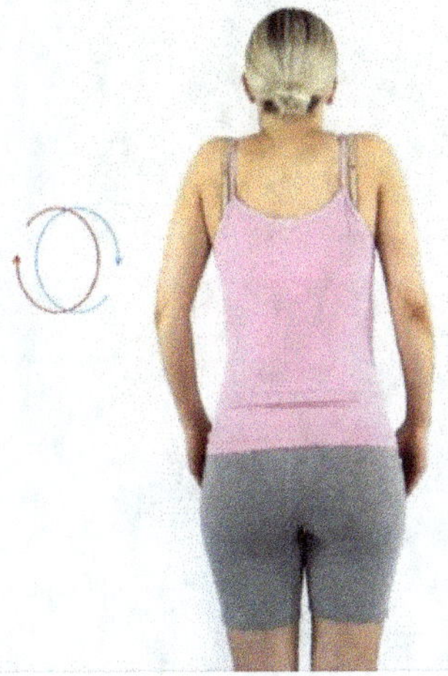

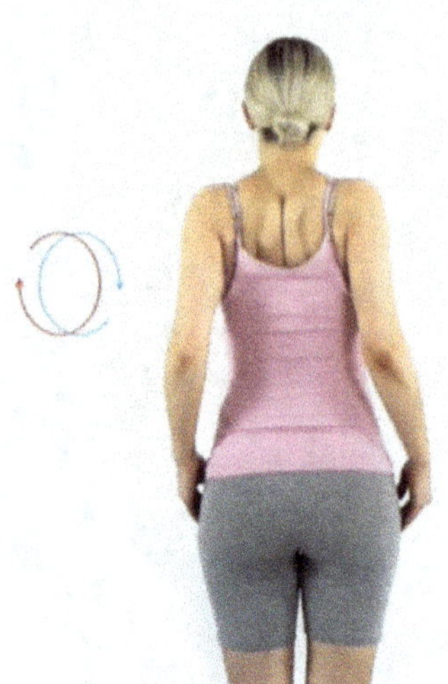

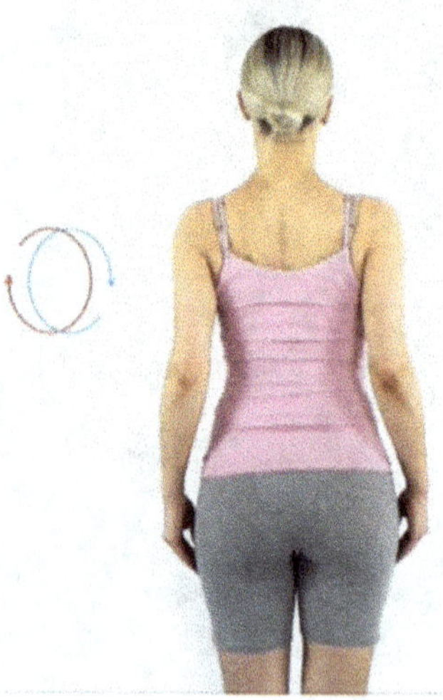

Step-by-Step Instructions:

1. Sit or stand comfortably with your arms relaxed at your sides.

2. Inhale and lift your shoulders towards your ears.

3. Exhale and roll your shoulders back and down.

4. Repeat ten times, then reverse the direction for another ten repetitions.

Tips:

Keep your movements smooth and controlled.

Focus on releasing tension from your shoulders.

Video guide: [Shoulder Roll Video]

4. Neck Release

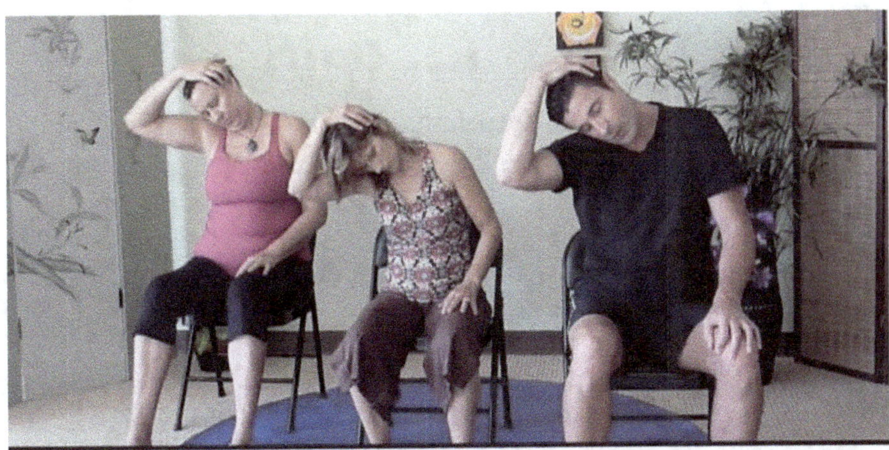

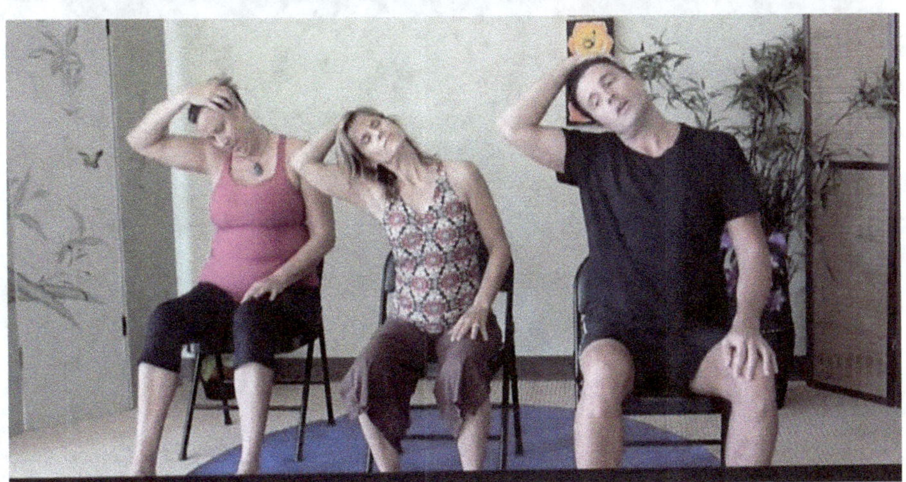

Step-by-Step Instructions:

1. Sit or stand comfortably with your back straight.
2. Gently tilt your head to the right, bringing your right ear towards your right shoulder.
3. Hold for a few breaths, feeling the stretch on the left side of your neck.
4. Repeat on the left side.
5. Perform five repetitions on each side.

Tips:

Move slowly to avoid straining your neck.

Use your breath to deepen the stretch.

Video guide: Neck Release Video

5. Spinal Twist

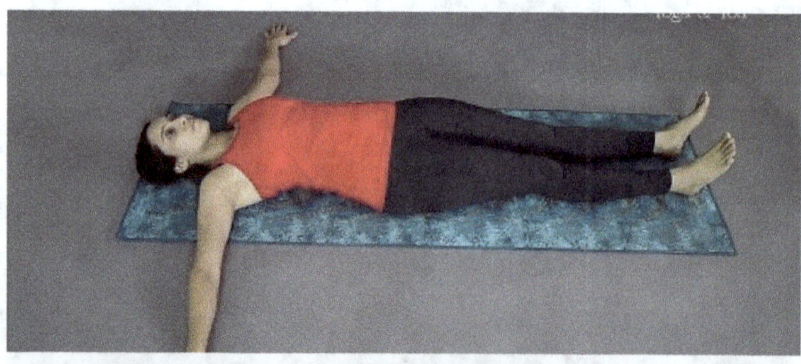

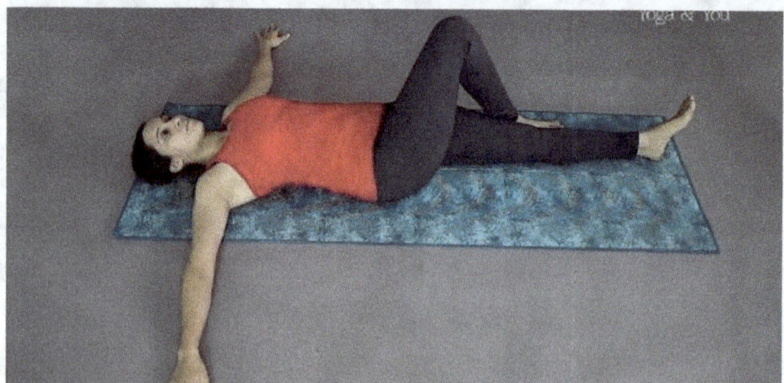

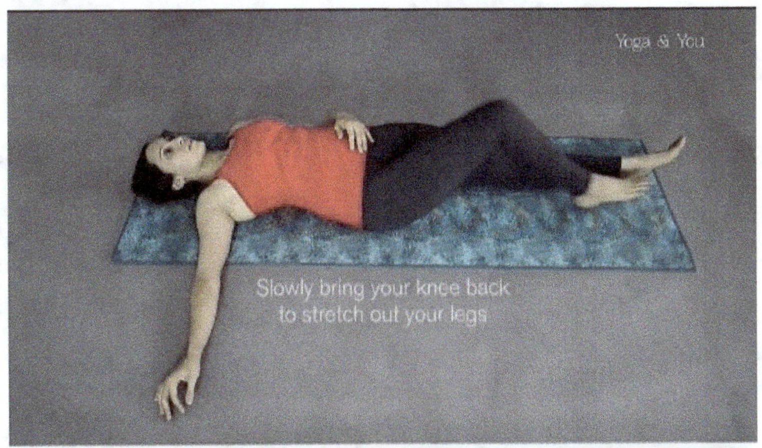
Yoga & You
Slowly bring your knee back
to stretch out your legs

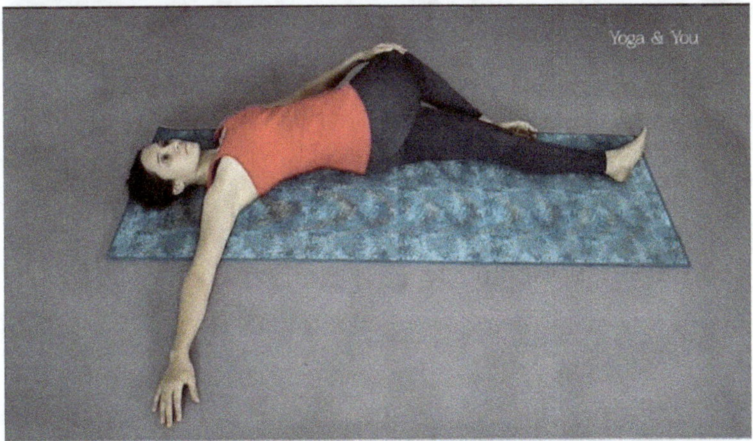
Yoga & You

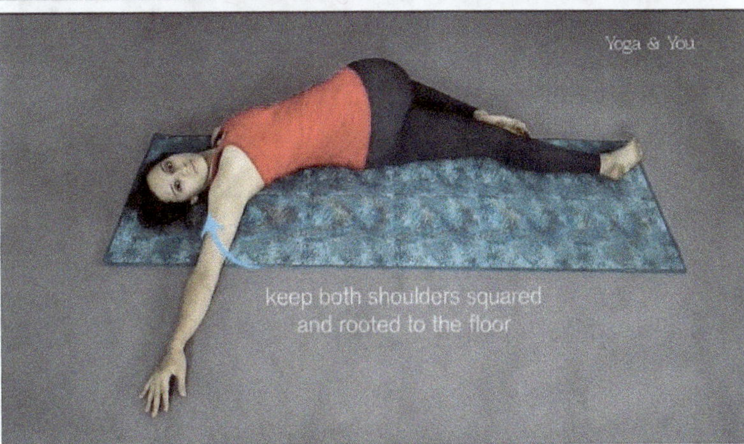
Yoga & You
keep both shoulders squared
and rooted to the floor

Step-by-Step Instructions:

1. Sit on the floor with your legs extended in front of you.

2. Bend your right knee and place your right foot on the outside of your left thigh.

3. Place your left hand on your right knee and your right hand behind you for support.

4. Inhale and lengthen your spine, then exhale and twist to the right.

5. Hold for a few breaths, then switch sides.

6. Perform five repetitions on each side.

Tips:

Keep your spine long and your movements gentle.

Use your breath to deepen the twist.

Video guide: [Spinal Twist Video](#)

6. Hip Opener

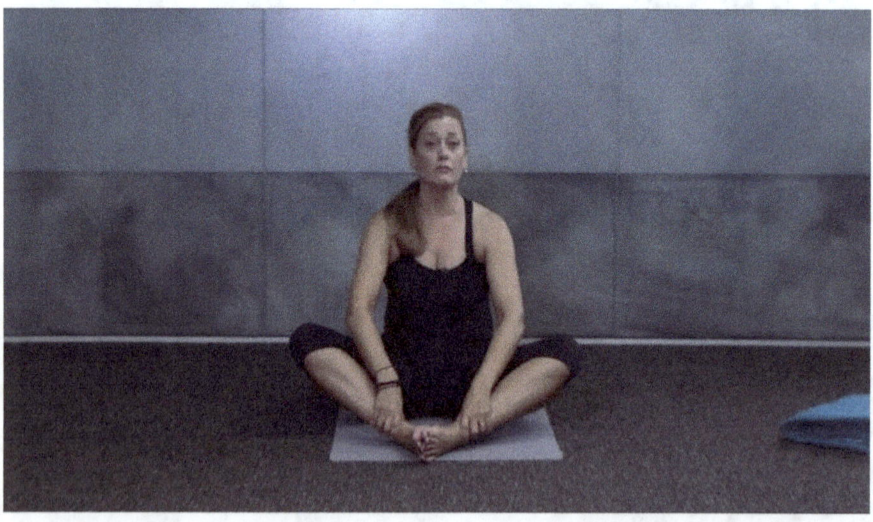

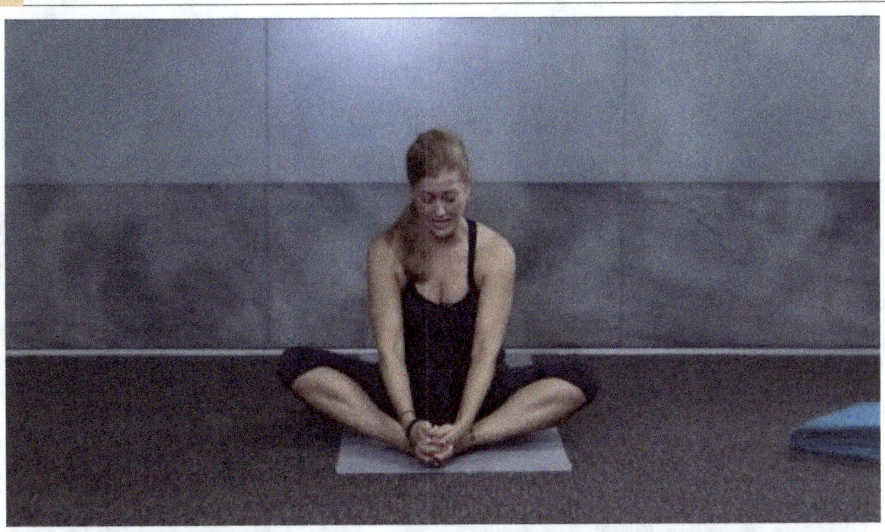

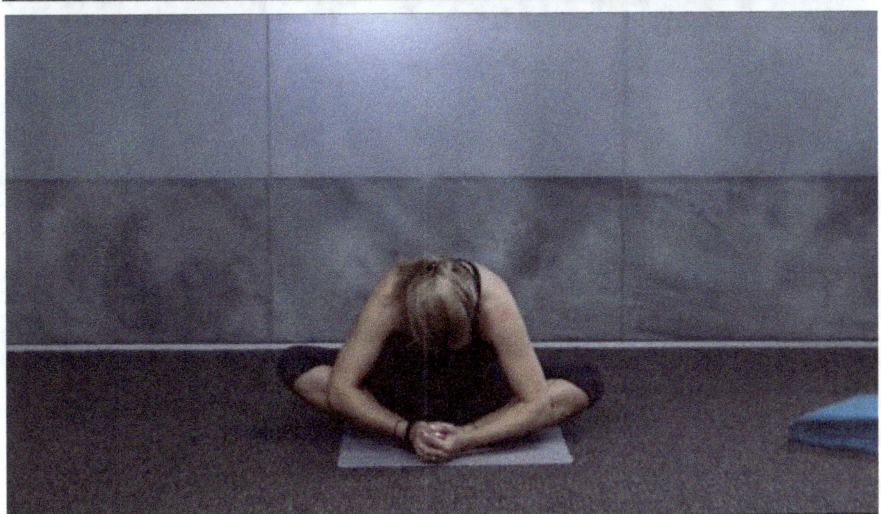

Step-by-Step Instructions:

1. Sit on the floor with your legs bent and feet together.

2. Hold your feet with your hands and gently press your knees towards the floor.

3. Inhale deeply and exhale as you gently press your knees down.

4. Hold for a few breaths, then release.

5. Perform ten repetitions.

Tips:

Avoid forcing your knees down; let gravity do the work.

Focus on the stretch in your hips and inner thighs.

Video guide: [Hip Opener Video](#)

7. Forward Bend

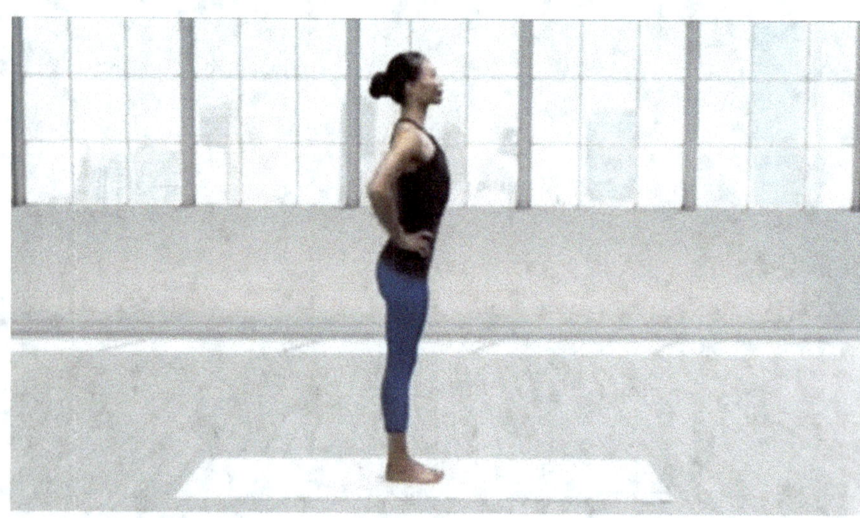

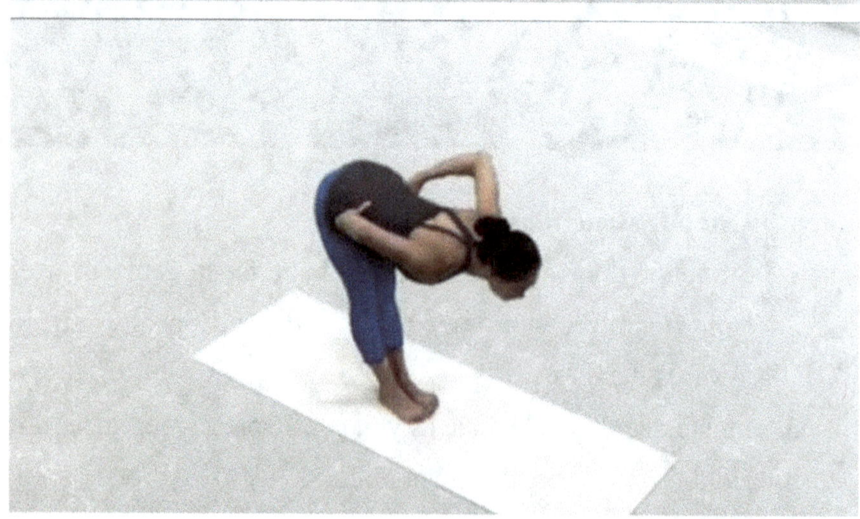

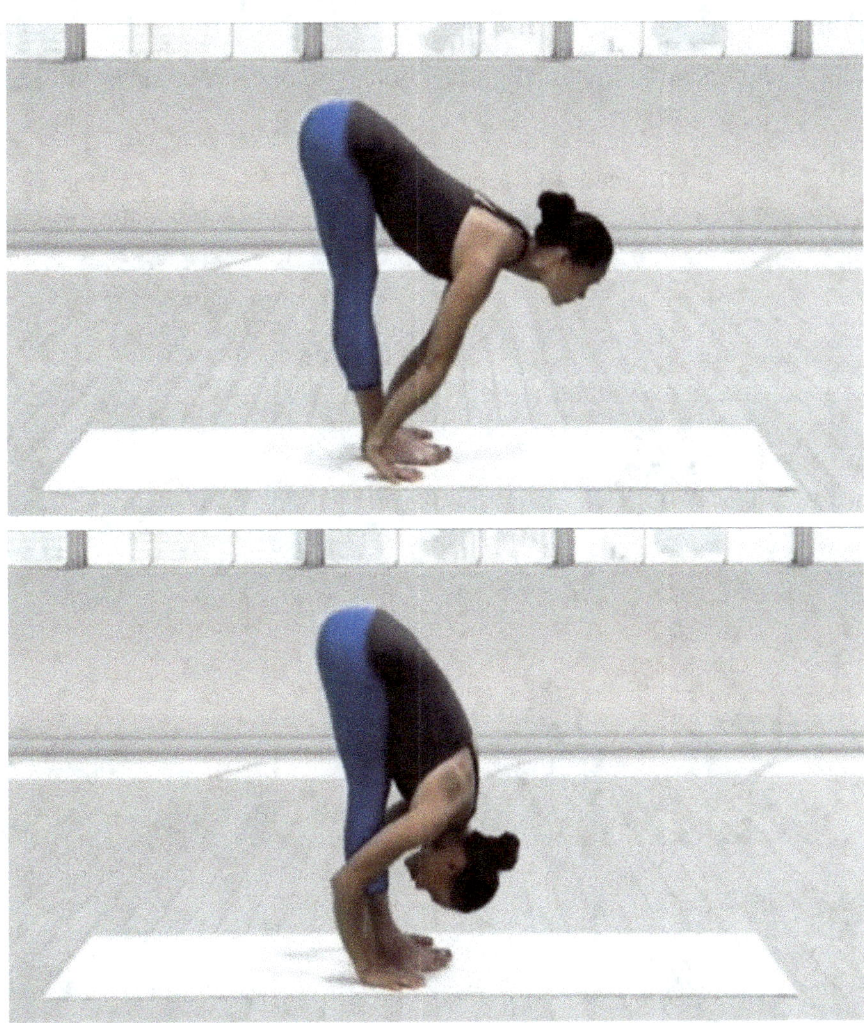

Step-by-Step Instructions:

1. Stand with your feet hip-width apart.

2. Inhale and reach your arms overhead.

3. Exhale and bend forward from your hips, letting your arms and head hang down.

4. Hold for a few breaths, then slowly rise back up.

5. Perform ten repetitions.

Tips:

Keep your knees slightly bent to avoid straining your lower back.

Use your breath to deepen the stretch.

Video guide: [Forward Bend Video](#)

8. Ankle Circles

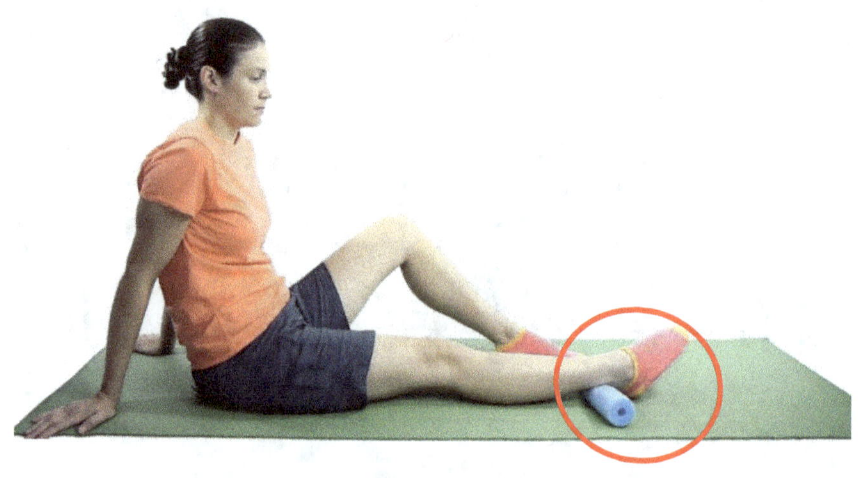

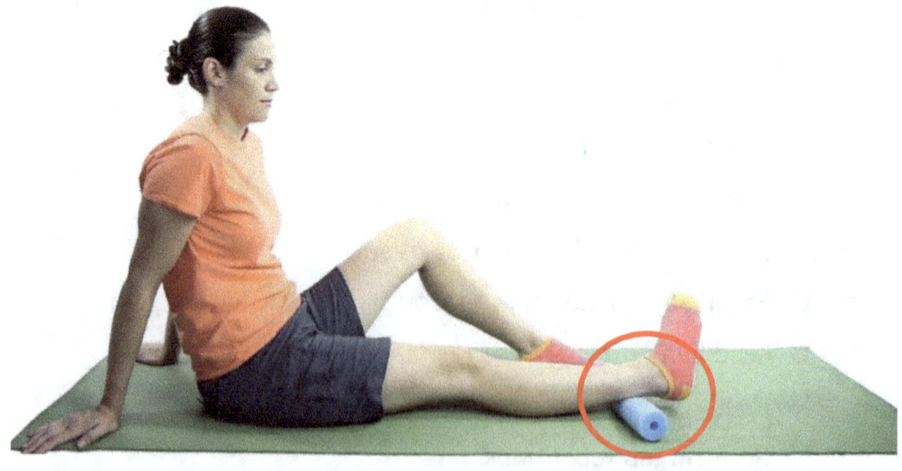

Step-by-Step Instructions:

1. Sit comfortably with your legs extended in front of you.

2. Lift your right leg and draw circles with your ankle.

3. Perform ten circles in one direction, then switch directions.

4. Repeat with the left ankle.

Tips:

Keep your movements slow and controlled.

Focus on the mobility in your ankles.

Video guide: Ankle Circles Video

9. Wrist Flexor Stretch

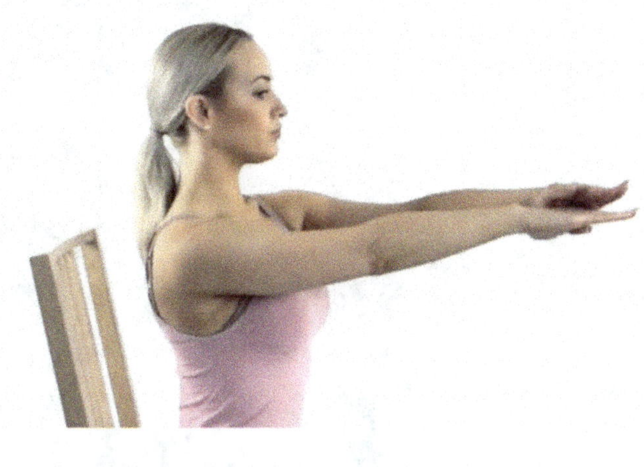

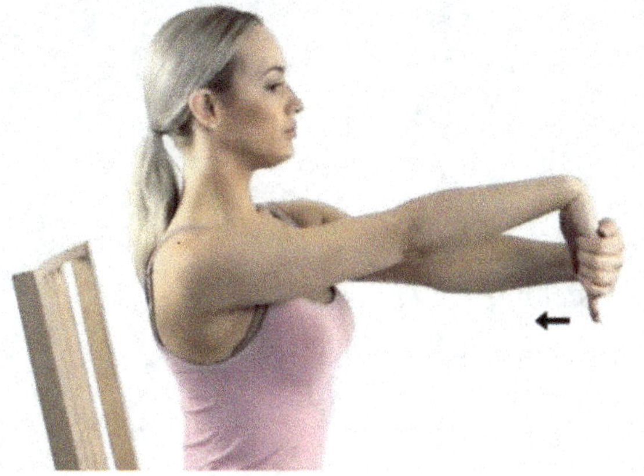

Step-by-Step Instructions:

1. Extend your right arm in front of you with your palm facing up.
2. Use your left hand to pull your right fingers back towards your body gently.
3. Hold for a few breaths, feeling the stretch in your forearm.
4. Repeat on the left side.
5. Perform five repetitions on each side.

Tips:

Move gently to avoid overstretching.

Use your breath to deepen the stretch.

Video guide: Wrist Flexor Stretch Video

10. Chest Opener

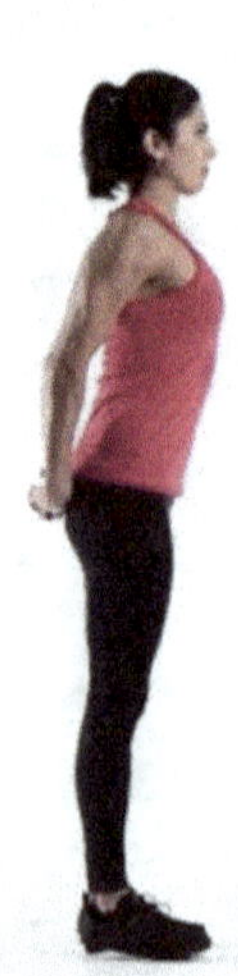

Step-by-Step Instructions:

1. Stand with your feet hip-width apart.
2. Clasp your hands behind your back.

3. Inhale and lift your chest, pulling your shoulders back.

4. Hold for a few breaths, then release.

5. Perform ten repetitions.

Tips:

Keep your movements slow and controlled.

Focus on opening your chest and releasing tension in your shoulders.

Video guide: Chest Opener Video

Tips for Maintaining Consistency and Motivation

1. **Set Realistic Goals:** Start with small, achievable goals to build confidence and momentum.

2. **Create a Routine:** Schedule regular practice sessions and stick to them. Consistency is key to seeing progress.

3. **Track Your Progress:** Keep a journal to document your practice, noting any improvements or challenges.

4. **Stay Positive:** Focus on the benefits and enjoy the process. Celebrate your achievements, no matter how small.

5. **Find a community:** Join a class or online group for support and motivation. Sharing your journey with others can be inspiring.

Visual Aids

Detailed Exercise Illustrations and Photographs

Here are illustrations and photographs for each exercise to help you visualize the movements. [Note: Images would be included here in the actual book or provided as links.]

Video Links for Guided Sessions

To further assist you, here are some video links to guided sessions for each exercise:

1. **Pelvic Tilt:** Pelvic Tilt Video
2. **Cat-Cow Stretch:** Cat-Cow Stretch Video
3. **Shoulder Roll:** Shoulder Roll Video
4. **Neck Release:** Neck Release Video
5. **Spinal Twist:** Spinal Twist Video
6. **Hip Opener:** Hip Opener Video
7. **Forward Bend:** Forward Bend Video
8. **Ankle Circles:** Ankle Circles Video
9. **Wrist Flexor Stretch:** Wrist Flexor Stretch Video
10. **Chest Opener:** Chest Opener Video

These simple routines and exercises, along with visual aids and guided sessions, provide a comprehensive foundation for your somatic practice. By following these steps and maintaining consistency, you'll enhance your body awareness, reduce tension, and improve your overall well-being.

CHAPTER 4: DEEPENING YOUR PRACTICE

Intermediate Techniques

As you advance in your somatic practice, you will build on foundational exercises and introduce more complex movements and sequences. These intermediate techniques will help deepen your body awareness, enhance flexibility, and improve overall physical and emotional well-being.

Intermediate Routines

1. Dynamic Bridge

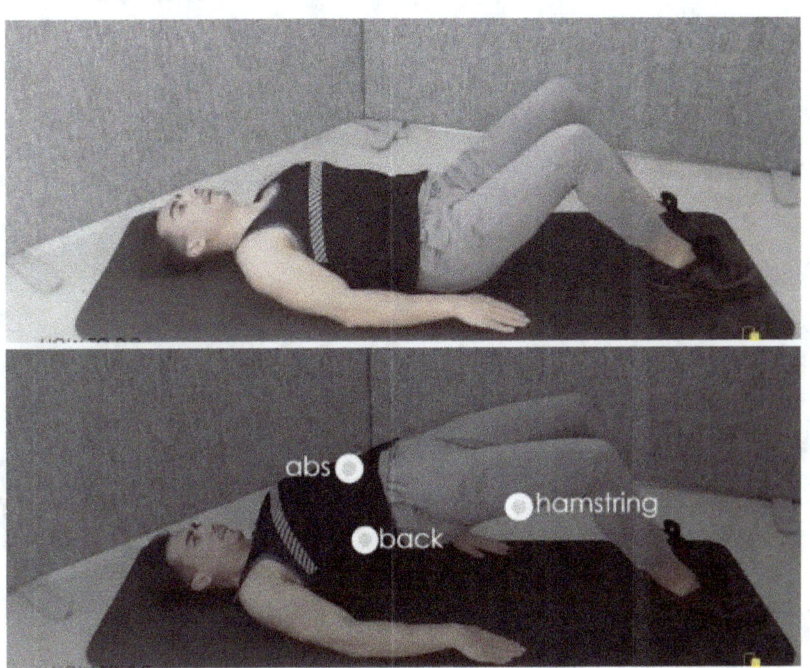

Step-by-Step Instructions:

1. Lie on your back with your knees bent and feet flat on the floor, hip-width apart.
2. Place your arms by your sides, palms facing down.
3. Inhale and lift your hips towards the ceiling, creating a straight line from your knees to your shoulders.
4. Exhale and slowly lower your hips back to the floor.
5. Repeat 15 times, focusing on the movement of your spine and hips.

Tips:

Engage your core and glutes to lift your hips.

Move slowly and with control.

Video guide: **Dynamic Bridge Video**

2. Seated Forward Fold with Twist

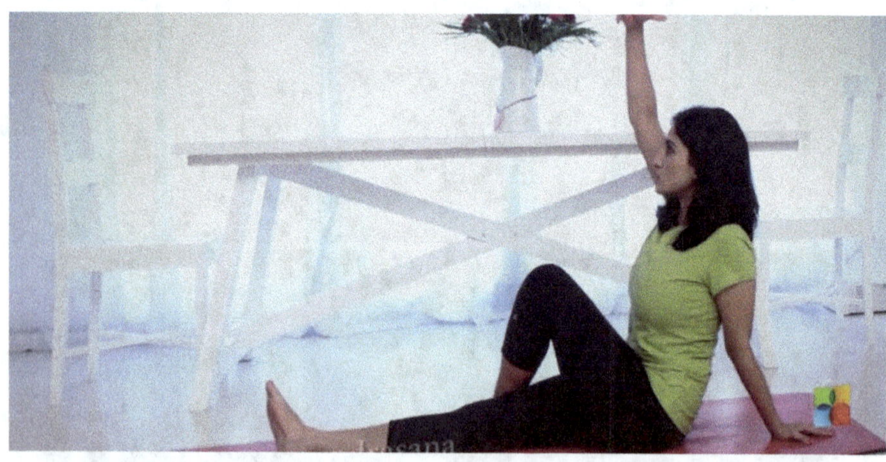

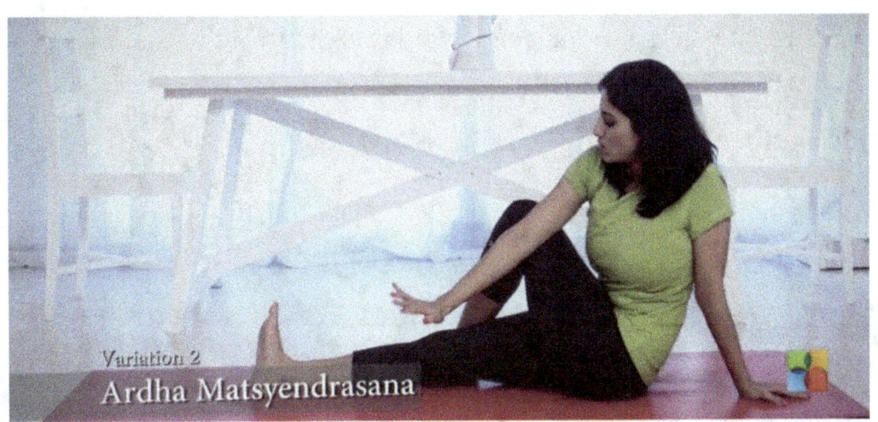

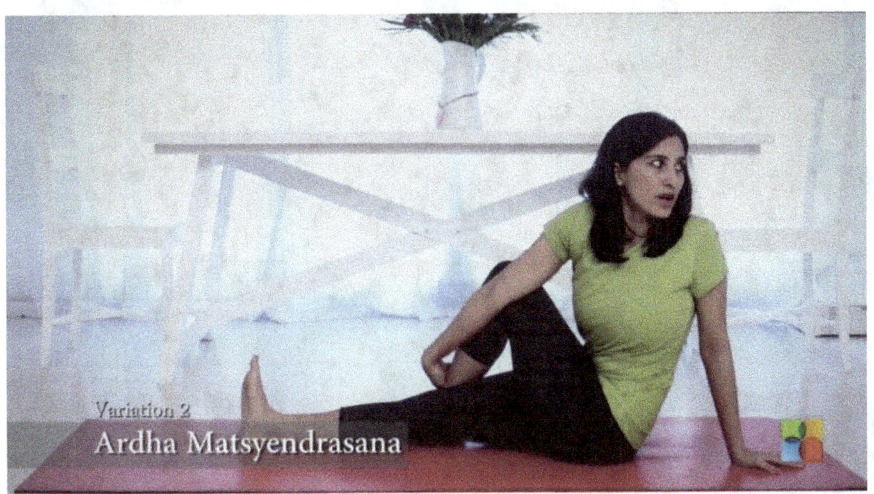

Step-by-Step Instructions:

1. Sit with your legs extended straight in front of you.

2. Inhale and lengthen your spine.

3. Exhale and fold forward from your hips, reaching for your toes.

4. Inhale and twist your torso to the right, placing your left hand on your right knee and your right hand behind you.

5. Hold for a few breaths, then return to the forward fold.

6. Repeat on the left side.

7. Perform ten repetitions on each side.

Tips:

Keep your spine long and avoid rounding your back.

Use your breath to deepen the stretch.

Video guide: [Forward Fold with Twist Video](#)

3. Side Plank

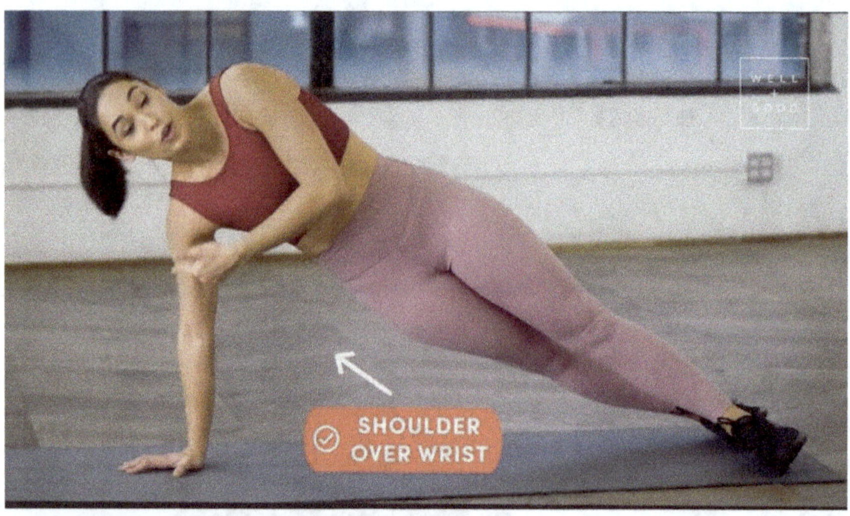

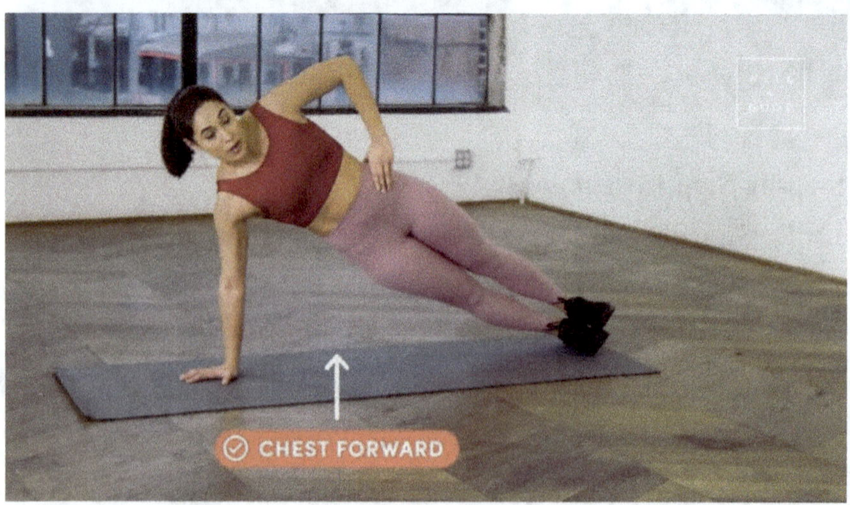

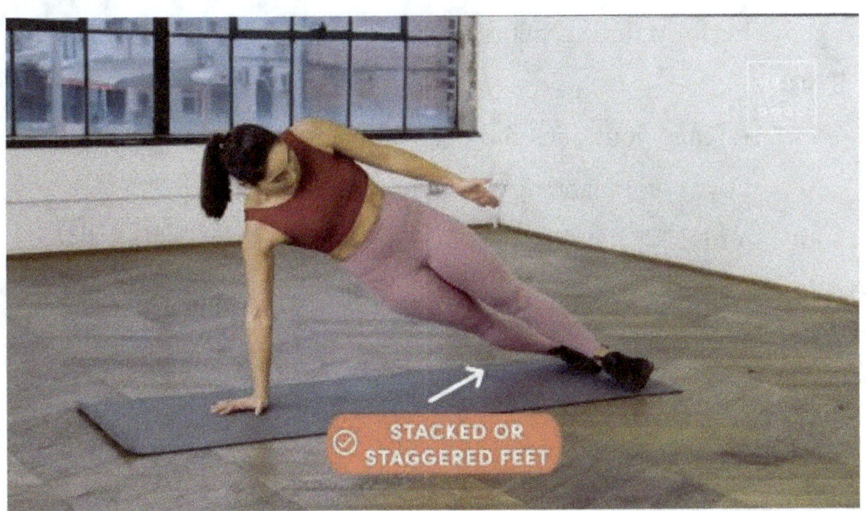

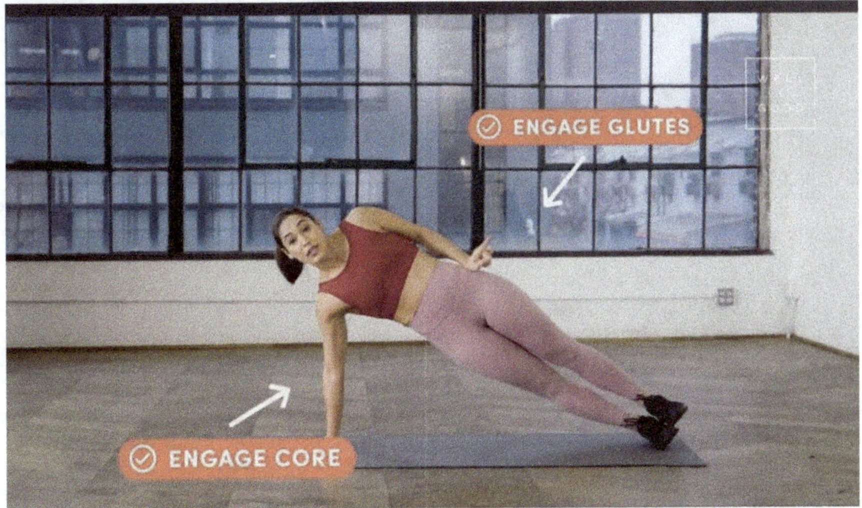

Step-by-Step Instructions:

1. Start in a plank position with your hands directly under your shoulders.

2. Shift your weight onto your right hand and the outer edge of your right foot.

3. Stack your left foot on top of your right and lift your left arm towards the ceiling, creating a straight line from your head to your feet.

4. Hold for 30 seconds, then switch sides.

5. Perform three repetitions on each side.

Tips:

Engage your core and keep your body in a straight line.

Focus on balancing and maintaining stability.

Video guide: [Side Plank]

4. Pigeon Pose with Forward Fold

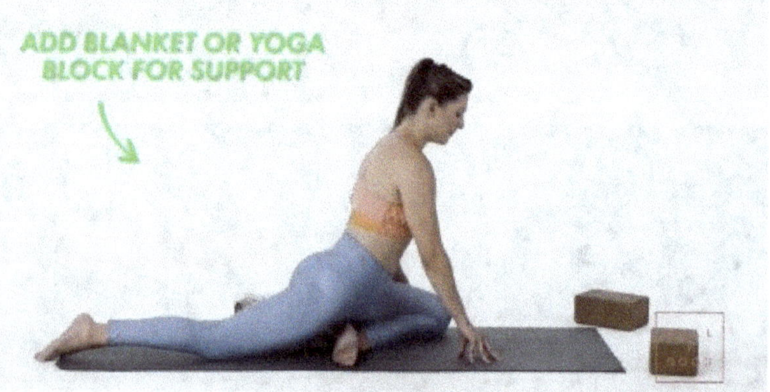

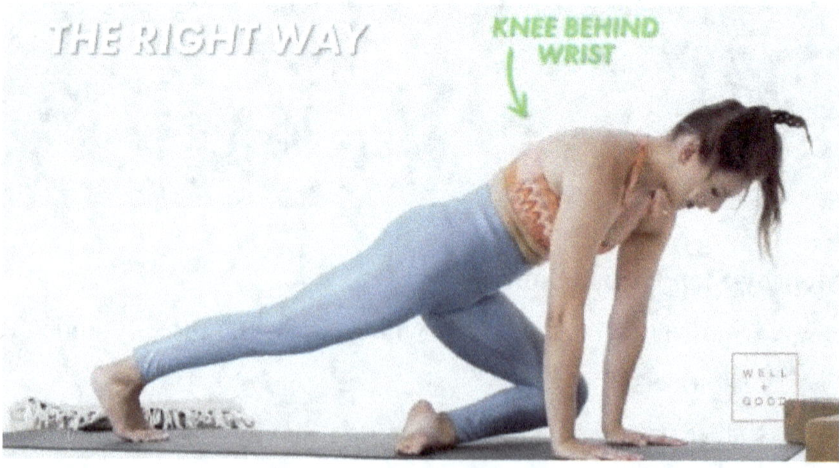

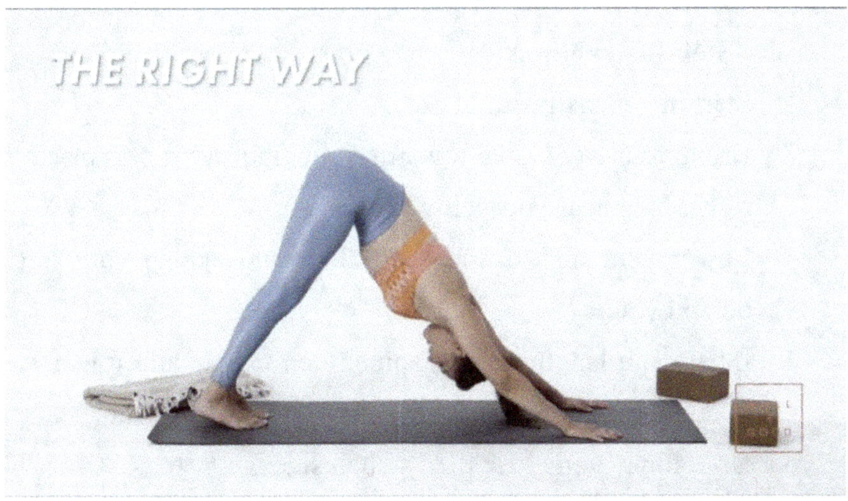
THE RIGHT WAY

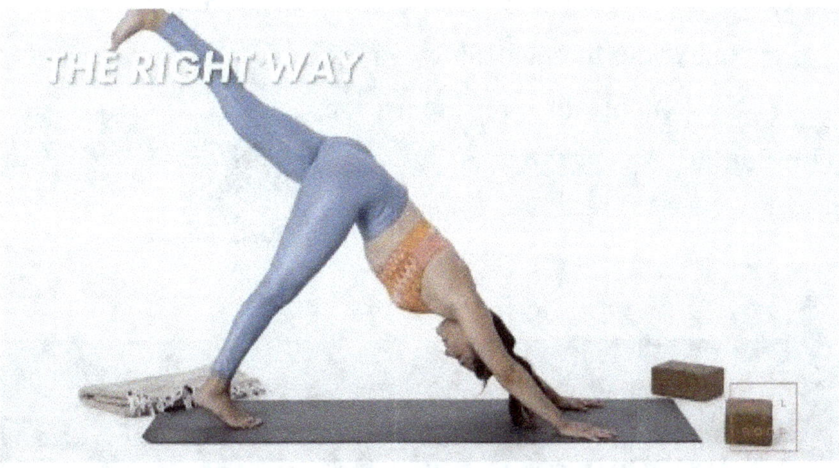
THE RIGHT WAY

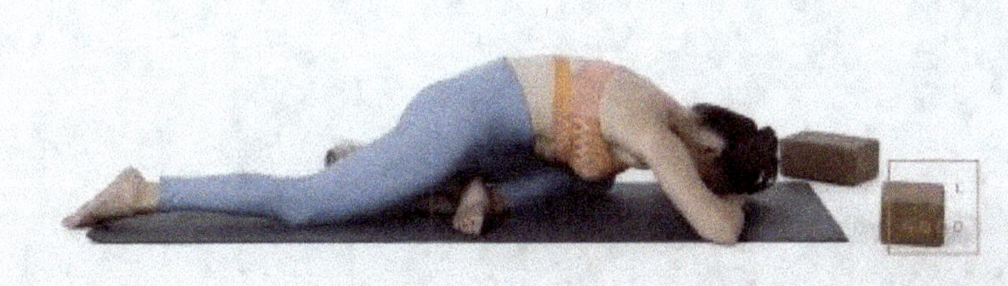

Step-by-Step Instructions:

1. Start in a plank position.
2. Bring your right knee towards your right wrist and place your right ankle near your left wrist.
3. Lower your hips towards the floor and extend your left leg behind you.
4. Inhale and lengthen your spine, then exhale and fold forward over your right leg.
5. Hold for 1-2 minutes, then switch sides.

Tips:

Relax your hips and allow gravity to deepen the stretch.

Use your breath to release tension.

Video guide: Pigeon Pose

5. Reverse Tabletop

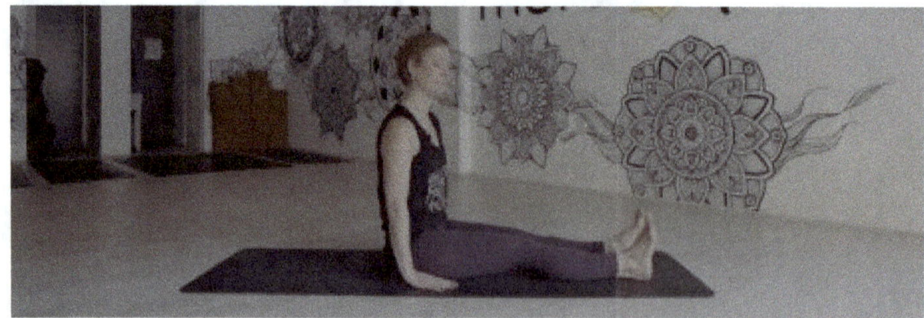

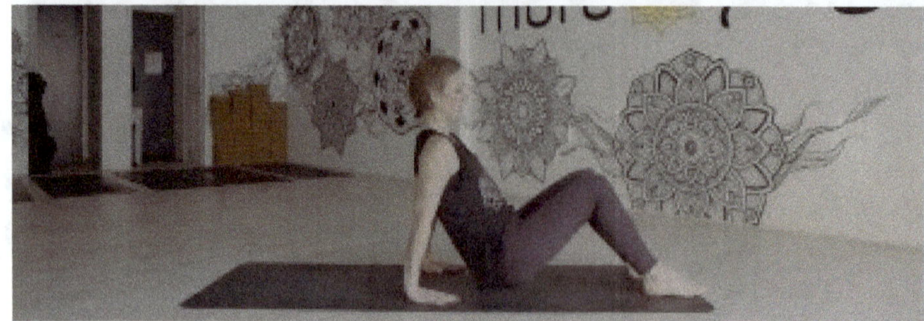

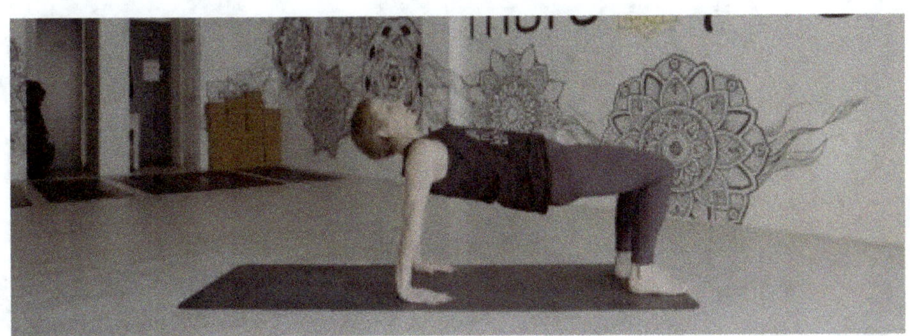

Step-by-Step Instructions:

1. Sit with your legs bent and feet flat on the floor, hip-width apart.
2. Place your hands behind you with your fingers pointing towards your feet.
3. Inhale and lift your hips towards the ceiling, creating a straight line from your knees to your shoulders.
4. Hold for a few breaths, then slowly lower your hips back to the floor.
5. Repeat 15 times.

Tips:

Engage your core and glutes to lift your hips.

Keep your neck relaxed and gaze towards the ceiling.

Video guide: [Reverse Tabletop Video](Reverse%20Tabletop%20Video)

6. Warrior III

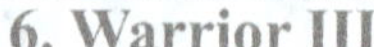

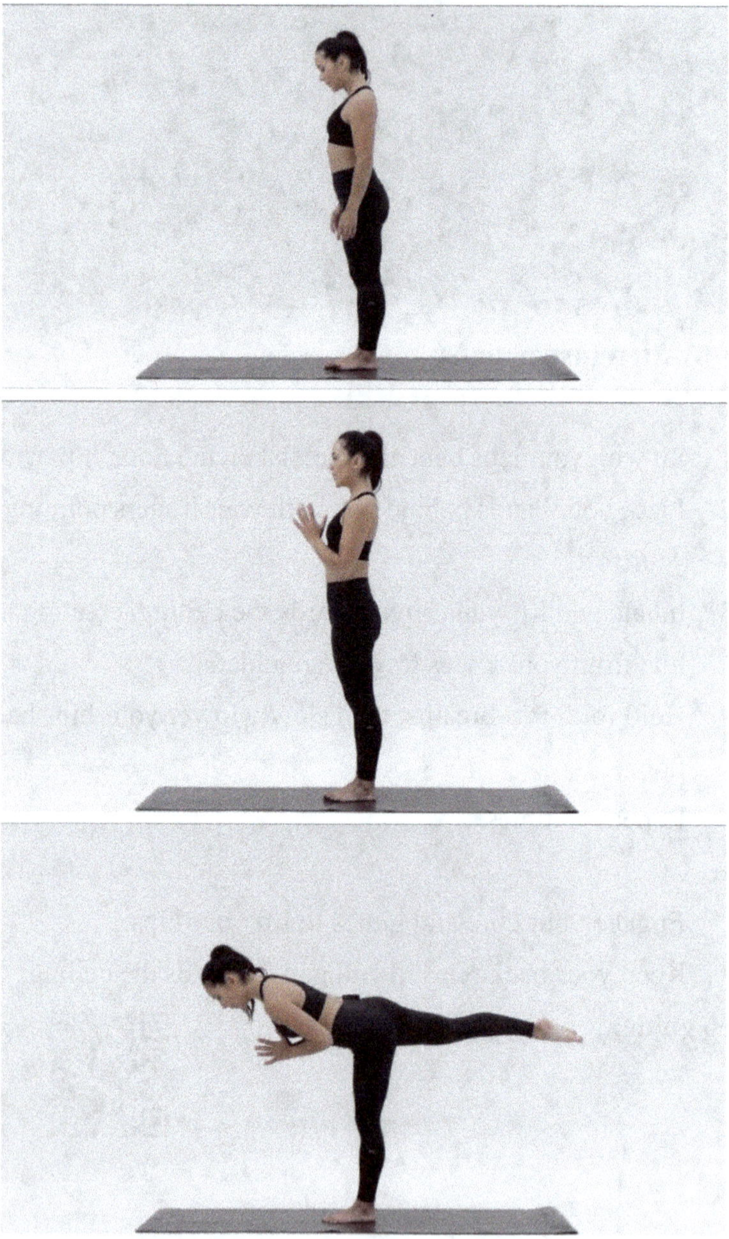

Step-by-Step Instructions:

1. Stand with your feet hip-width apart.

2. Shift your weight onto your right foot and lift your left leg behind you, keeping it straight.

3. Extend your arms forward, creating a straight line from your

fingertips to your left heel.

4. Hold for 30 seconds, then switch sides.

5. Perform three repetitions on each side.

Tips:

Engage your core and keep your body in a straight line.

Focus on balancing and maintaining stability.

Video guide: [Warrior III Video]

7. Eagle Pose

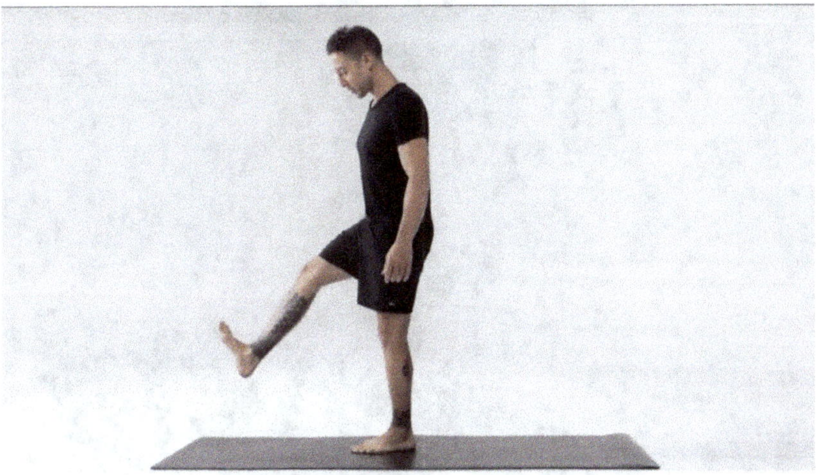

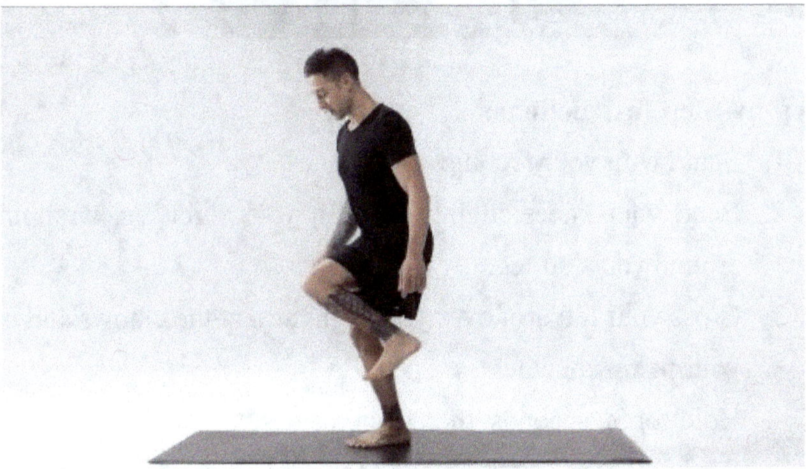

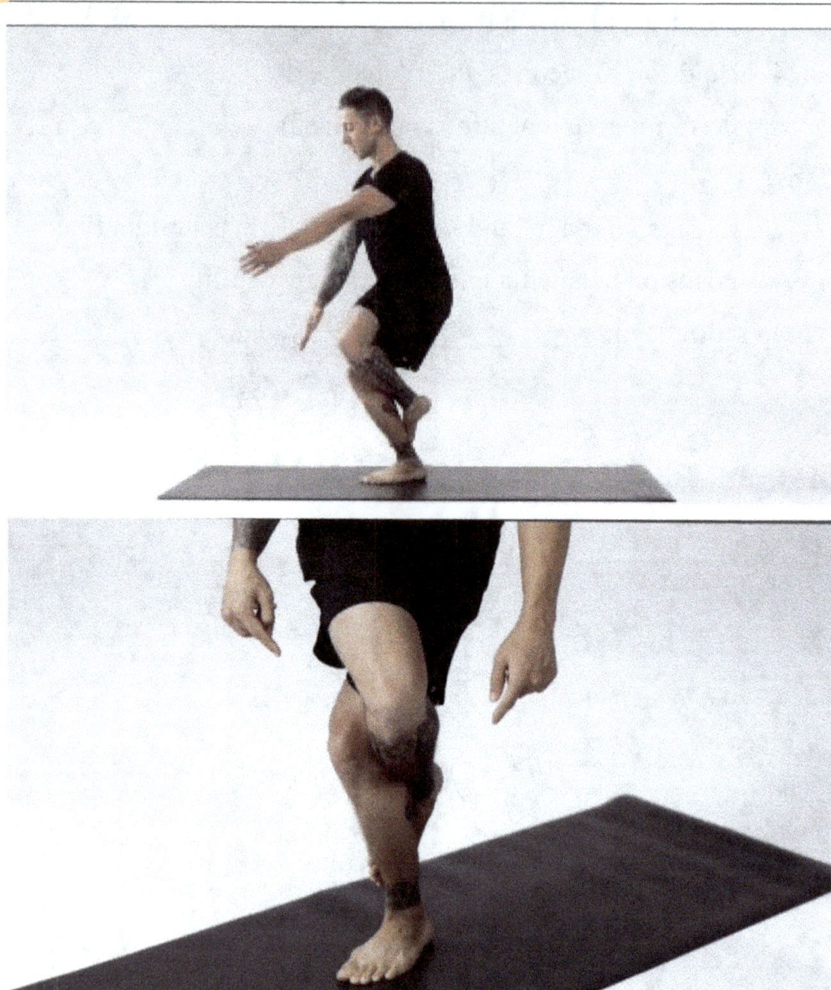

Step-by-Step Instructions:

1. Stand with your feet hip-width apart.

2. Bend your knees slightly and lift your right leg, wrapping it around your left leg.

3. Cross your left arm over your right arm at the elbows and bring your palms together.

4. Hold for 30 seconds, then switch sides.

5. Perform three repetitions on each side.

Tips:

Engage your core and maintain balance.

Focus on the stretch in your shoulders and hips.

Video guide: Eagle Pose Video

8. Reclining Bound Angle Pose

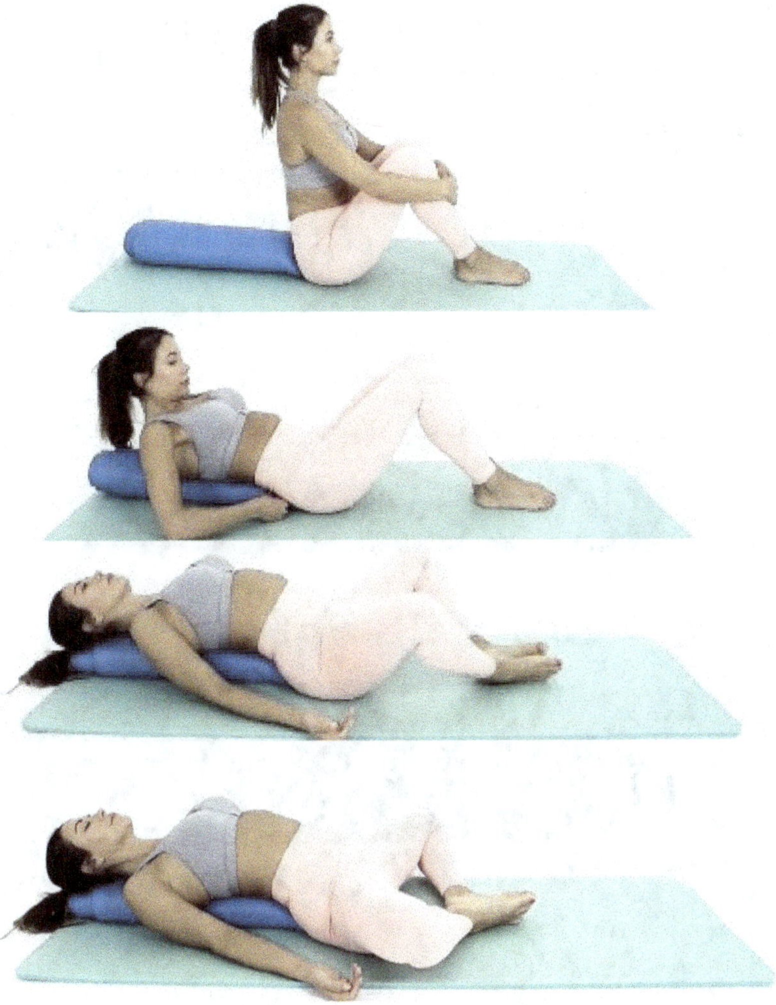

Step-by-Step Instructions:

1. Lie on your back with your knees bent and feet flat on the floor.

2. Bring the soles of your feet together and let your knees fall open to the sides.

3. Place your hands on your lower abdomen.

4. Hold for 1-2 minutes, focusing on your breath.

Tips:

Relax your hips and allow gravity to deepen the stretch.

Use your breath to release tension.

Video guide: **Reclining Bound Angle Pose Video**

9. Bow Pose

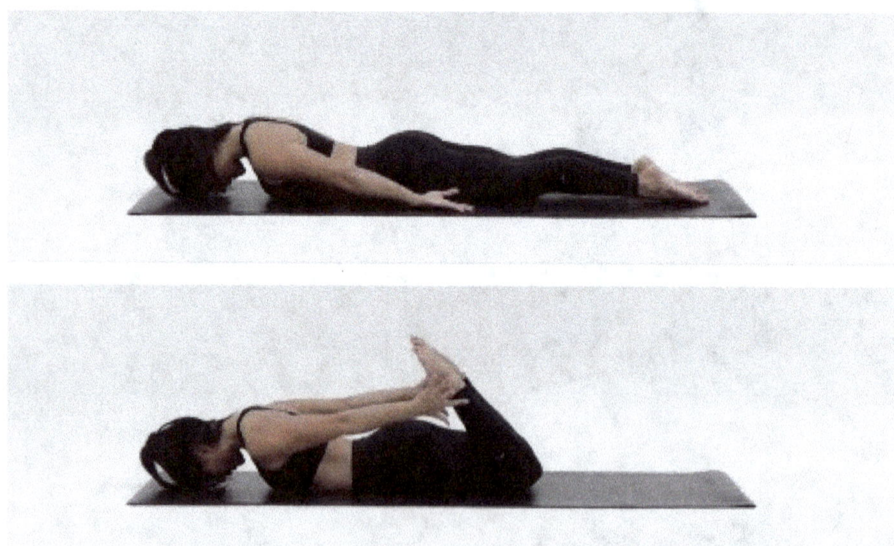

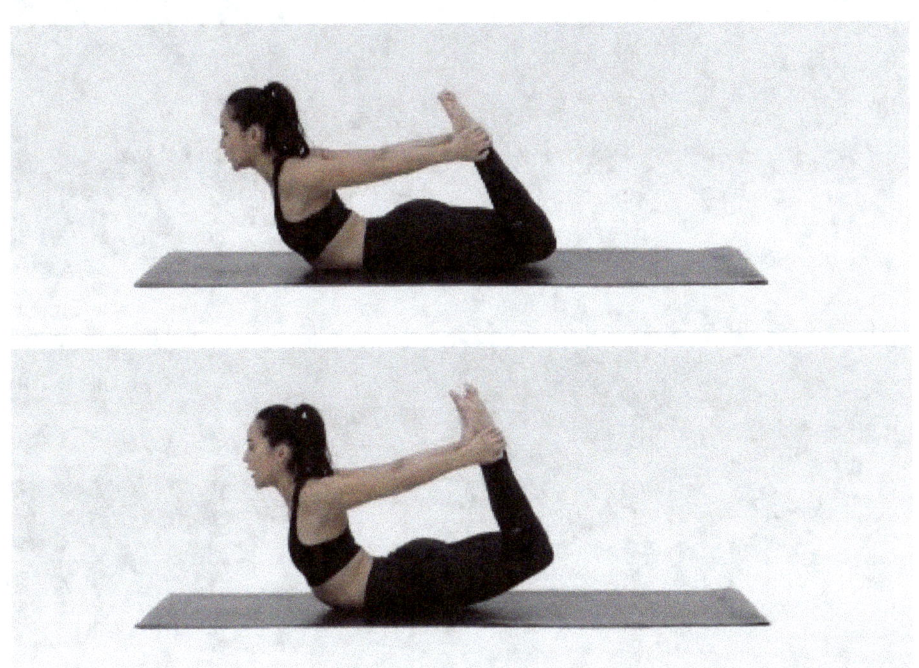

Step-by-Step Instructions:

1. Lie on your stomach with your legs extended and arms by your sides.
2. Bend your knees and reach back to grab your ankles.
3. Inhale and lift your chest and legs off the floor, pulling your ankles towards the ceiling.
4. Hold for 30 seconds, then release.
5. Perform five repetitions.

Tips:

Engage your core and keep your neck relaxed.

Focus on the stretch in your chest and thighs.

Video guide: Bow Pose Video

10. Reclining Spinal Twist

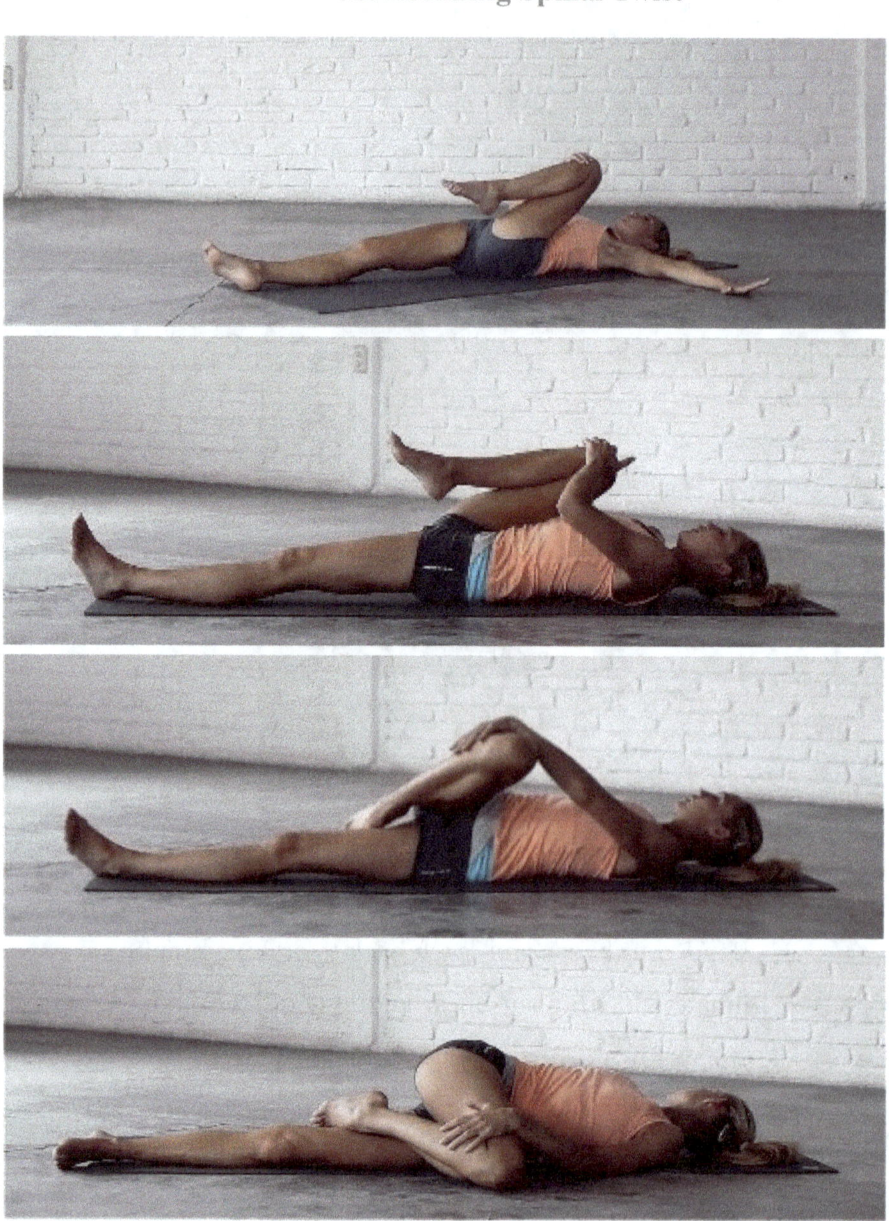

Step-by-Step Instructions:

1. Lie on your back with your legs extended.

2. Bend your right knee and bring it towards your chest.

3. Cross your right knee over to the left side of your body, extending your right arm to the side and looking towards your right hand.

4. Hold for 1-2 minutes, then switch sides.

Tips:

Relax your shoulders and allow your spine to twist naturally.

Use your breath to deepen the stretch.

Video guide: Spinal Twist Video

Overcoming Common Challenges

Handling Physical Discomfort and Mental Resistance

1. **Physical Discomfort:**

    o   **Listen to Your Body:** Pay attention to your body's signals and avoid pushing through pain. Discomfort is normal, but pain is a sign to stop and adjust.

    o   **Modify Exercises:** Use props like blocks, straps, or cushions to modify exercises and make them more comfortable.

    o   **Take Breaks:** Allow yourself to take breaks when needed. Resting is an important part of the practice.

2. **Mental Resistance:**

    o   **Stay Present:** Focus on your breath and the sensations in your body to stay present and mindful.

    o   **Set Realistic Goals:** Break down your practice into smaller, achievable goals to avoid feeling overwhelmed.

    o   **Be Patient:** Progress takes time. Be patient with yourself and celebrate small achievements.

Adjusting Exercises to Fit Individual Needs

1. **Personalize Your Practice:**

   o **Adaptations:** Modify exercises to suit your body and its current capabilities. For example, use a chair for balance or reduce the range of motion.

   o **Listen to Your Body:** Pay attention to how your body feels and adjust your practice accordingly. Each day may be different, and it's important to honor your body's needs.

Visual Aids

Progressive Exercise Diagrams

Diagrams will illustrate the progression from basic to intermediate exercises, showing the key movements and muscle engagement.

Comparative Charts Showing Progressions

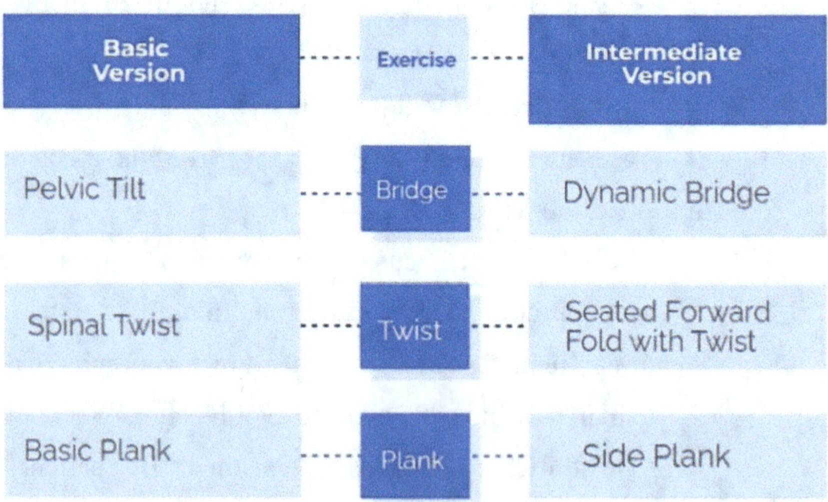

Video Links for Guided Sessions

1. **Dynamic Bridge:** Dynamic Bridge Video
2. **Seated Forward Fold with Twist:** Forward Fold with Twist Video
3. **Side Plank:** Side Plank
4. **Pigeon Pose with Forward Fold:** Pigeon Pose
5. **Reverse Tabletop:** Reverse Tabletop Video
6. **Warrior III:** Warrior III Video
7. **Eagle Pose:** Eagle Pose Video
8. **Reclining Bound Angle Pose:** Reclining Bound Angle Pose Video
9. **Bow Pose:** Bow Pose Video
10. **Reclining Spinal Twist:** Spinal Twist Video

These intermediate routines and exercises, along with visual aids and guided sessions, will help deepen your somatic practice. By building on foundational exercises and introducing more complex movements, you can enhance your body awareness, flexibility, and overall well-being.

CHAPTER 5: INTEGRATING SOMATIC EXERCISES INTO DAILY LIFE

Making It a Habit

Incorporating somatic exercises into your daily routine can be a transformative experience, leading to improved physical and mental well-being. Here are practical tips and strategies to make somatic exercises a regular part of your life.

Tips for Incorporating Exercises into Your Routine

1. **Start Small:**
   - Begin with just a few minutes each day to avoid feeling overwhelmed. Gradually increase the duration as you become more comfortable.
   - Example: Dedicate 5-10 minutes each morning to a simple somatic routine like breathing exercises and gentle stretches.

2. **Consistency is Key:**
   - Set a specific time each day for your practice. Consistency helps in forming a habit.
   - Example: Practice somatic exercises every evening before bed to help unwind and prepare for restful sleep.

3. **Create a Dedicated Space:**
   - Designate a quiet and comfortable area in your home for

your somatic practice. This helps signal to your brain that it's time to focus on your exercises.

- o Example: Use a corner of your living room with a yoga mat, cushions, and calming décor.

4. **Integrate with Daily Activities:**
   - o Incorporate somatic exercises into your daily routine to make it feel less like an added task and more like a natural part of your day.
   - o Example: Practice mindful breathing while waiting in line or do shoulder rolls during work breaks.

5. **Use Reminders and Cues:**
   - o Set reminders on your phone or place sticky notes in visible areas to prompt you to practice.
   - o Example: Set a reminder to practice a short routine after lunch every day.

Combining Somatic Exercises with Daily Activities

1. **Morning Routine:**
   - o **Exercise:** Start your day with a body scan meditation while still in bed.
   - o **Integration:** As you brush your teeth, practice standing on one leg to improve balance and body awareness.

2. **Work Environment:**
   - o **Exercise:** Take breaks to do seated spinal twists and neck stretches.
   - o **Integration:** Practice mindful breathing while typing or attending meetings to stay calm and focused.

3. **Household Chores:**
   - o **Exercise:** Incorporate lunges or squats while cleaning or cooking.
   - o **Integration:** Practice hip circles while waiting for the

kettle to boil or for food to cook.

4. **Evening Wind-Down:**
   - **Exercise:** Perform a series of gentle stretches and deep breathing exercises before bed.
   - **Integration:** Practice diaphragmatic breathing while watching TV or reading.

Real-Life Applications

Using Somatic Exercises to Manage Stress, Improve Posture, and Enhance Overall Well-Being

1. **Managing Stress:**
   - **Technique:** Diaphragmatic Breathing
   - **Application:** Use this technique during stressful moments, such as before a presentation or after a hectic day, to calm the mind and body.

2. **Improving Posture:**
   - **Technique:** Shoulder Rolls and Cat-Cow Stretch
   - **Application:** Incorporate these exercises into your daily routine, especially if you spend long hours sitting, to alleviate tension and improve posture.

3. **Enhancing Overall Well-Being:**
   - **Technique:** Body Scan Meditation and Pelvic Tilt
   - **Application:** Regularly practice these exercises to increase body awareness, reduce chronic pain, and promote a sense of relaxation and well-being.

Visual Aids

Examples of Daily Integration Scenarios

1. **Morning Routine Integration:**
   - **Scenario:** Wake up, perform a body scan meditation, and then practice gentle stretching while preparing for the day.

2. **Work Break Integration:**
   - **Scenario:** Take a break every hour to do neck stretches and shoulder rolls at your desk.

3. **Evening Wind-Down Integration:**
   - **Scenario:** Incorporate deep breathing exercises and reclining bound angle pose before bed to relax and prepare for sleep.

Chapter 6: Advanced Somatic Practices

Exploring Advanced Techniques

In this chapter, we will delve into advanced somatic exercises that build upon foundational and intermediate techniques. These exercises are designed to challenge your body awareness, enhance your flexibility, and integrate complex movements for a comprehensive full-body practice.

Advanced Routines

1. Standing Balance Series

Step-by-Step Instructions:

1. **Tree Pose:**
   - Stand with your feet hip-width apart.
   - Shift your weight onto your left foot and place your right foot on the inside of your left thigh or calf (avoid the knee).
   - Bring your hands to the prayer position at your chest.
   - Hold for 30 seconds, then switch sides.

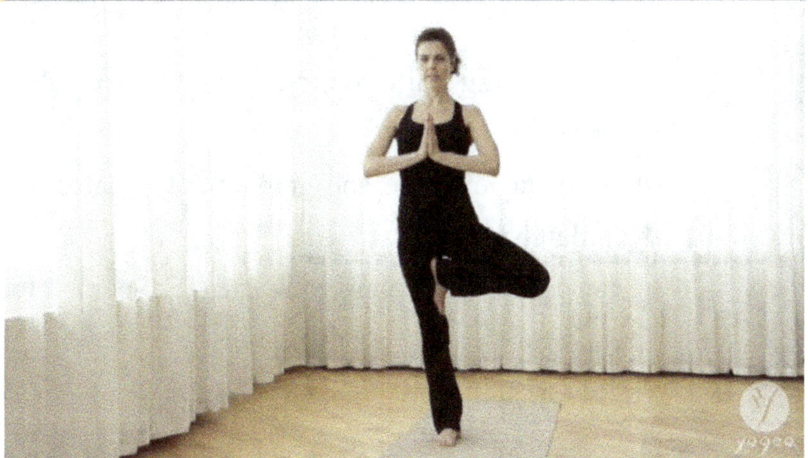

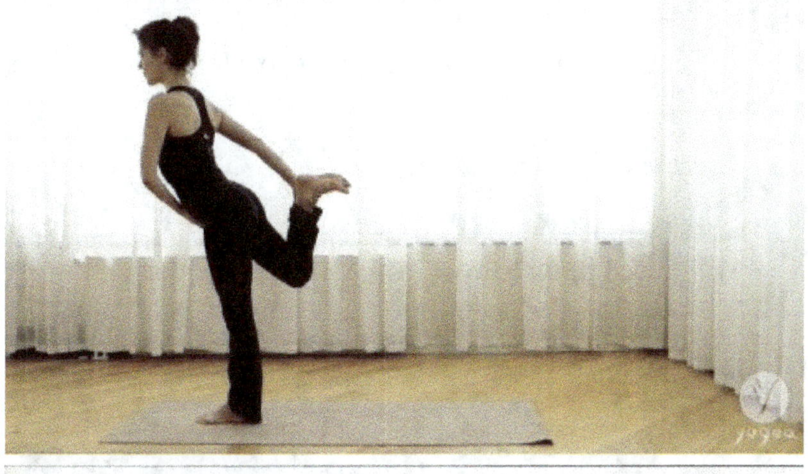

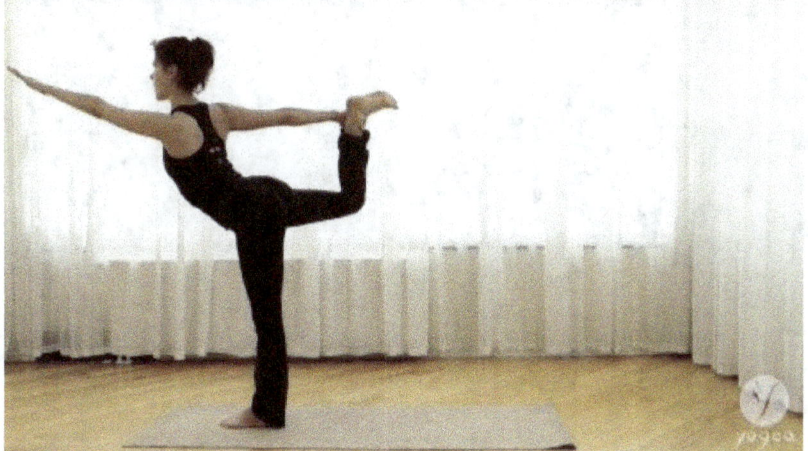

Dancer's Pose:

- o From standing, shift your weight onto your right foot.
- o Bend your left knee and grab your left ankle with your left hand.
- o Extend your right arm forward and kick your left foot back, lifting your leg and chest.
- o Hold for 30 seconds, then switch sides.

Tips:

Engage your core and focus on a fixed point to maintain balance.

Breathe deeply and steadily.

Video guide: Standing Balance Series Video

2. Advanced Spinal Twist

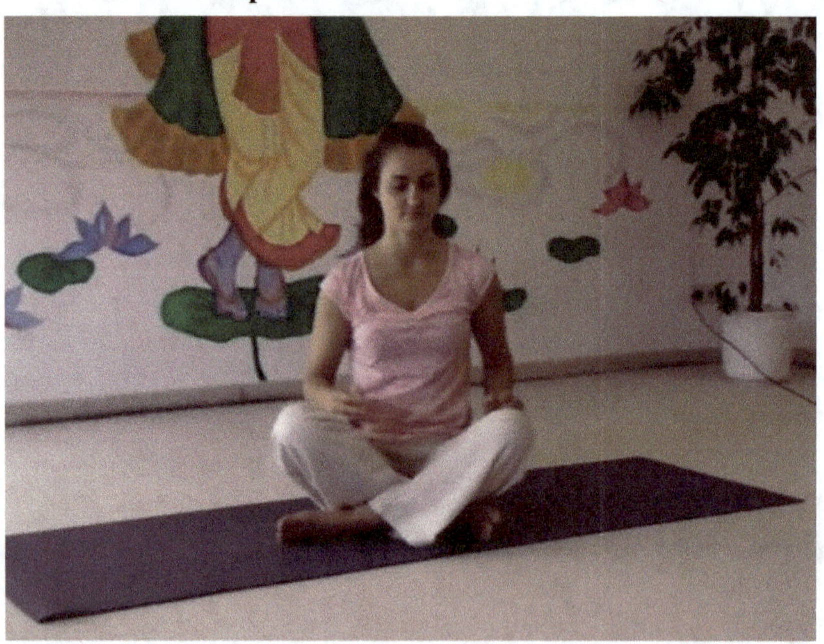

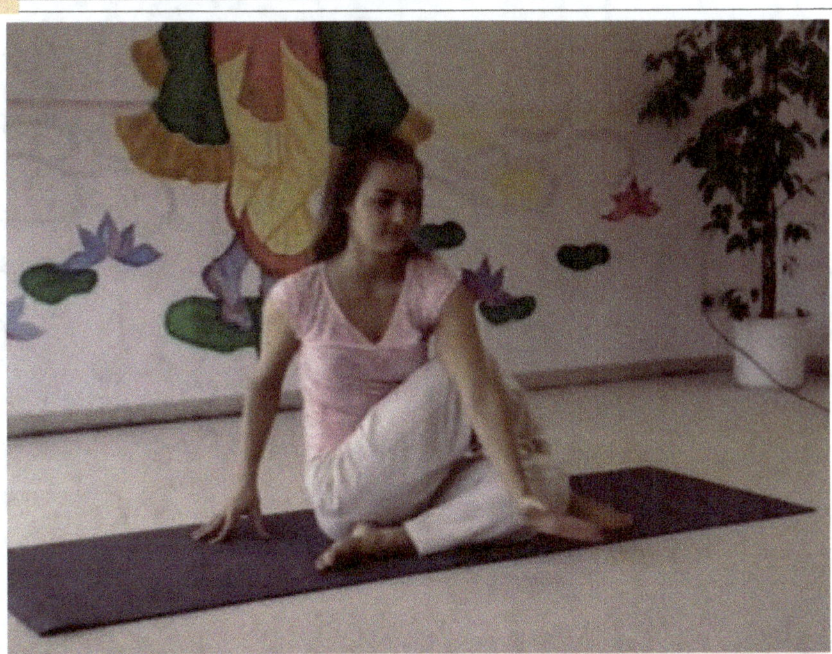

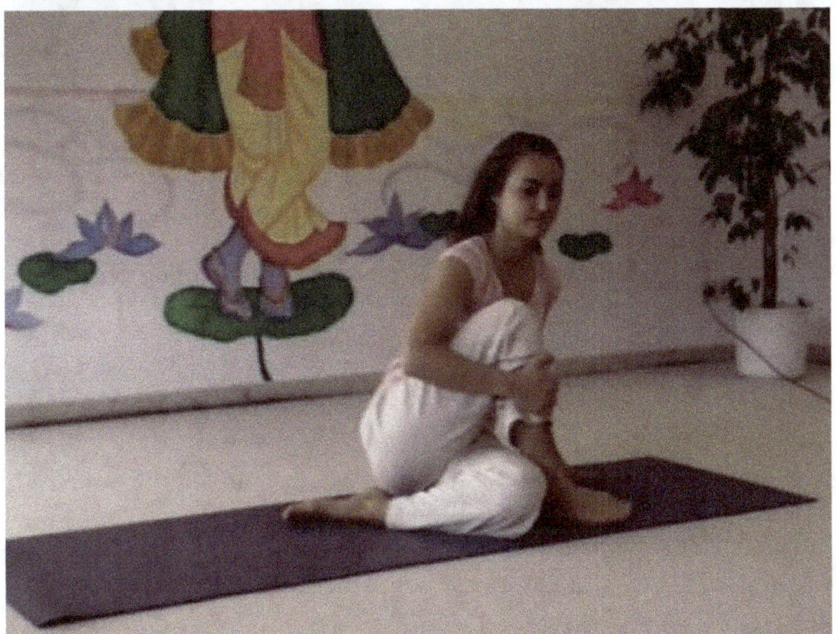

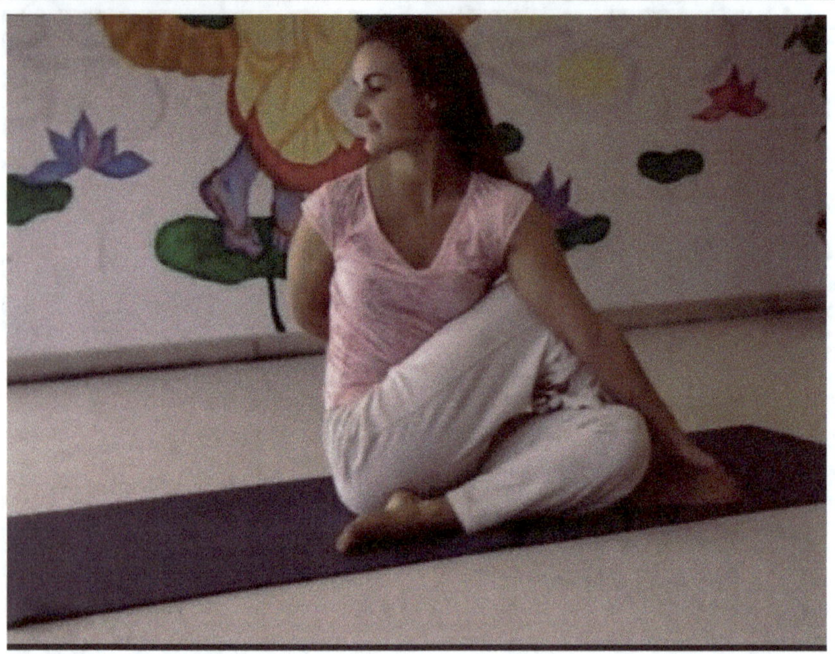

Step-by-Step Instructions:

1. Sit on the floor with your legs extended.
2. Bend your right knee and place your right foot on the outside of your left thigh.
3. Bend your left knee and bring your left foot near your right hip.
4. Place your right hand behind you for support.
5. Inhale, lengthen your spine, then exhale and twist to the right, hooking your left elbow on the outside of your right knee.
6. Hold for 1 minute, then switch sides.

Tips:

Keep your spine long and your movements controlled.

Use your breath to deepen the twist.

Video guide: [Advanced Spinal Twist Video](#)

3. Crow Pose

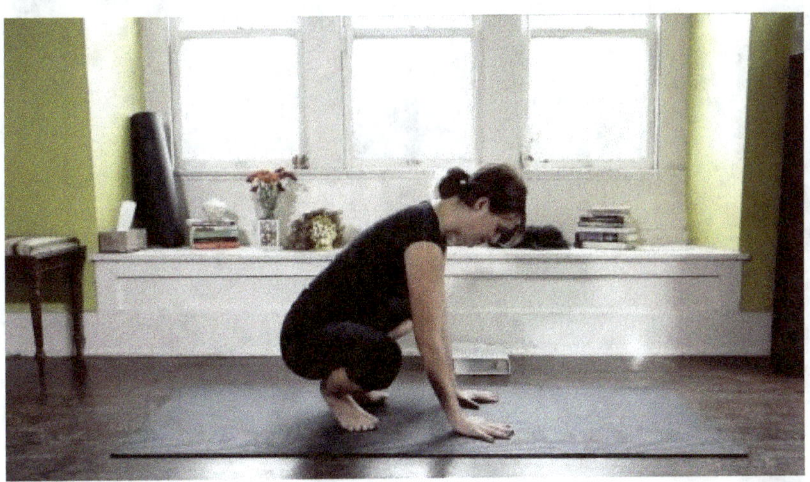

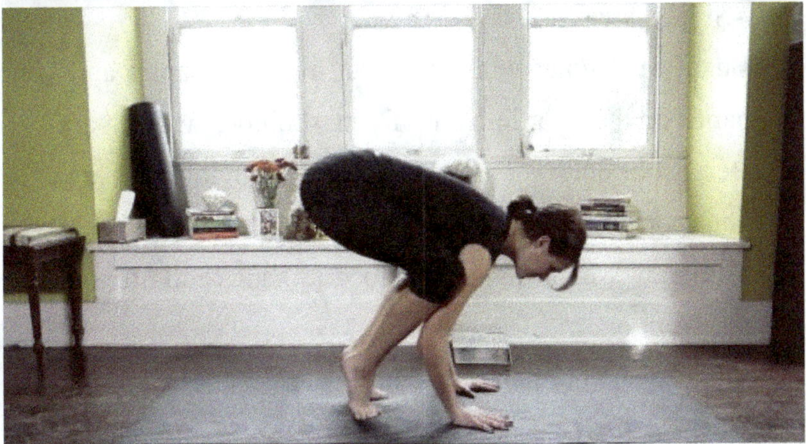

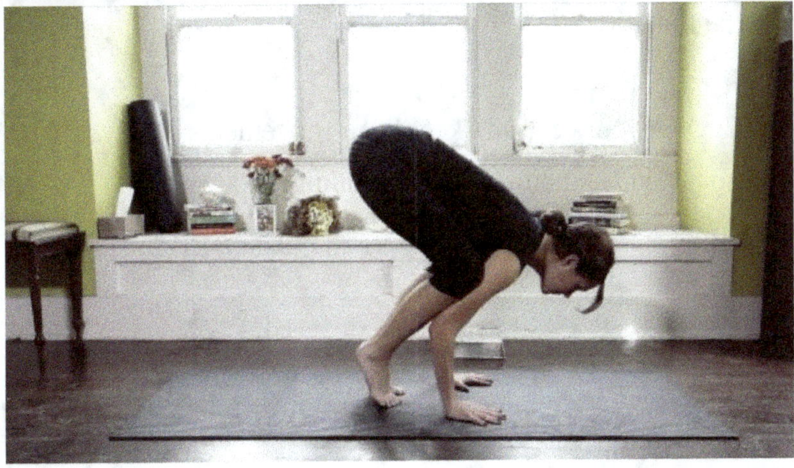

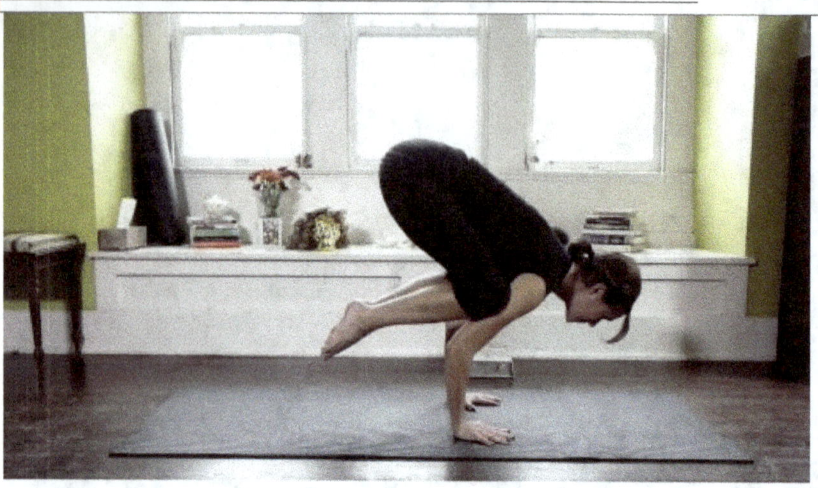

Step-by-Step Instructions:

1. Begin in a squat with your feet hip-width apart and your hands on the floor in front of you, shoulder-width apart.
2. Bend your elbows and lift your hips, bringing your knees to your upper arms.
3. Shift your weight forward onto your hands and lift your feet off the floor.
4. Balance on your hands, keeping your gaze forward.
5. Hold for 20-30 seconds, then slowly lower your feet back to the floor.

Tips:

Engage your core and keep your movements steady.

Focus on balancing and maintaining stability.

Video guide: Crow Pose Video

4. Pigeon Pose with Forward Fold and Arm Extension

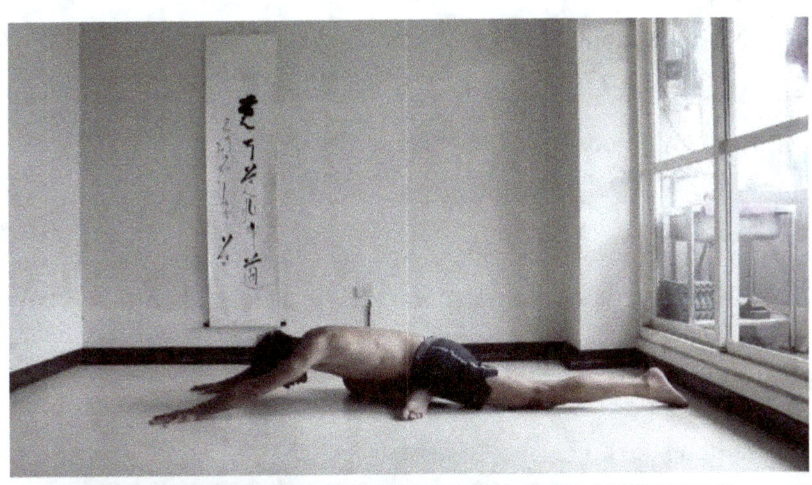

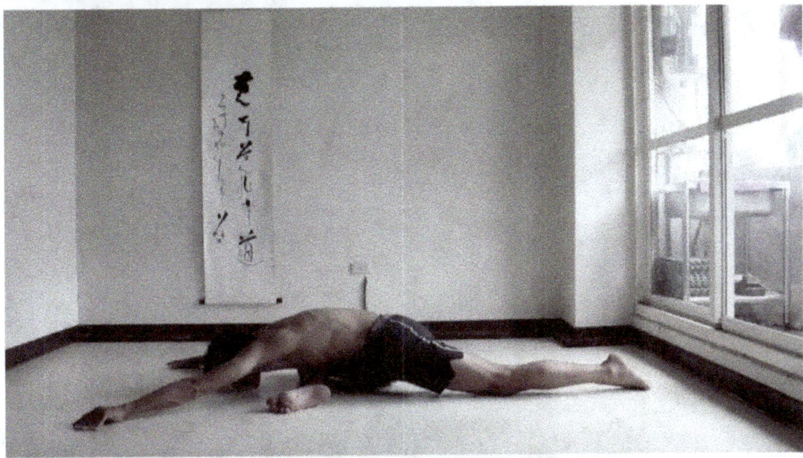

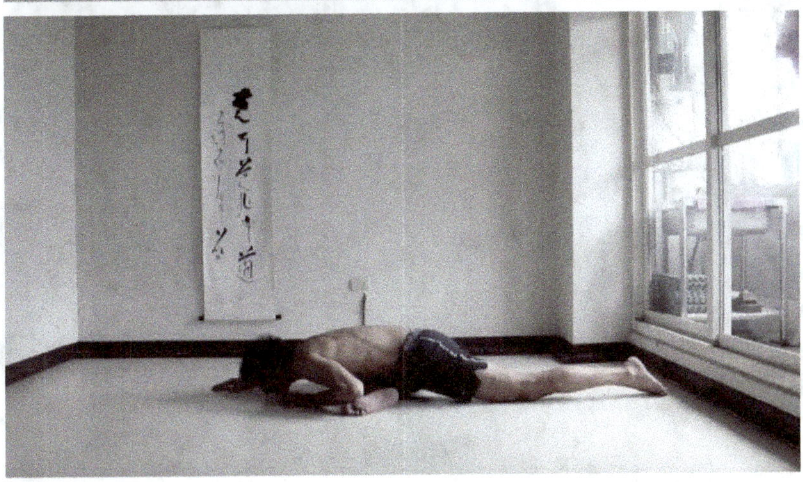

Step-by-Step Instructions:

1. Start in a plank position.
2. Bring your right knee towards your right wrist and place your right ankle near your left wrist.
3. Lower your hips towards the floor and extend your left leg behind you.
4. Inhale, lengthen your spine, then exhale and fold forward over your right leg.
5. Extend your arms forward and hold for 1-2 minutes, then switch sides.

Tips:

Relax your hips and allow gravity to deepen the stretch.

Use your breath to release tension.

Video guide: Pigeon pose

5. Warrior III with Arm Variations

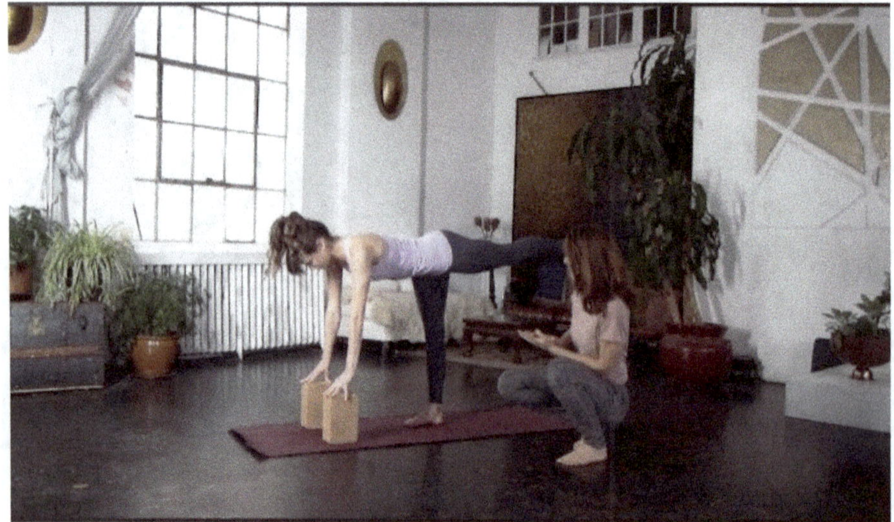

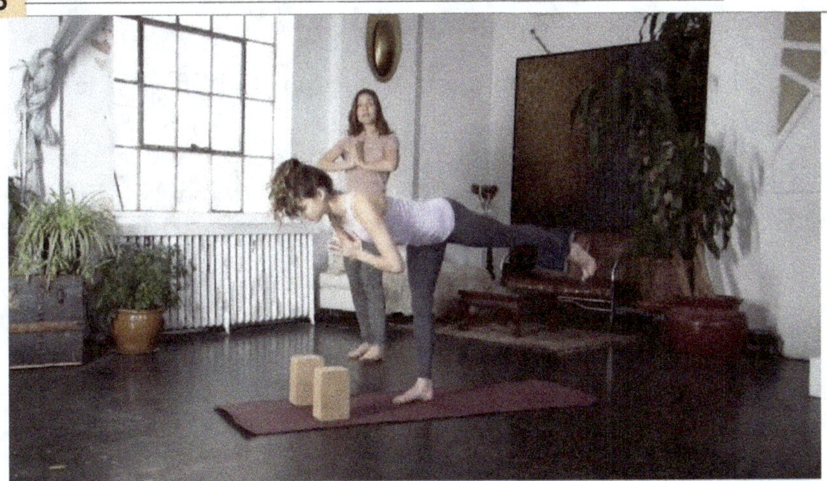

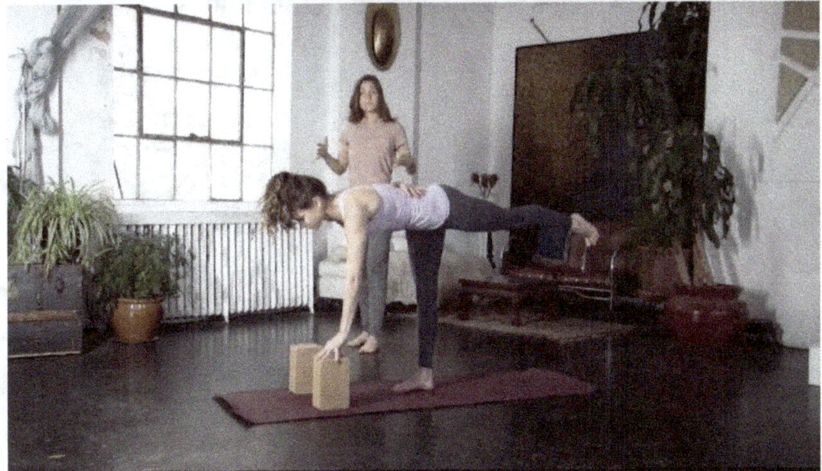

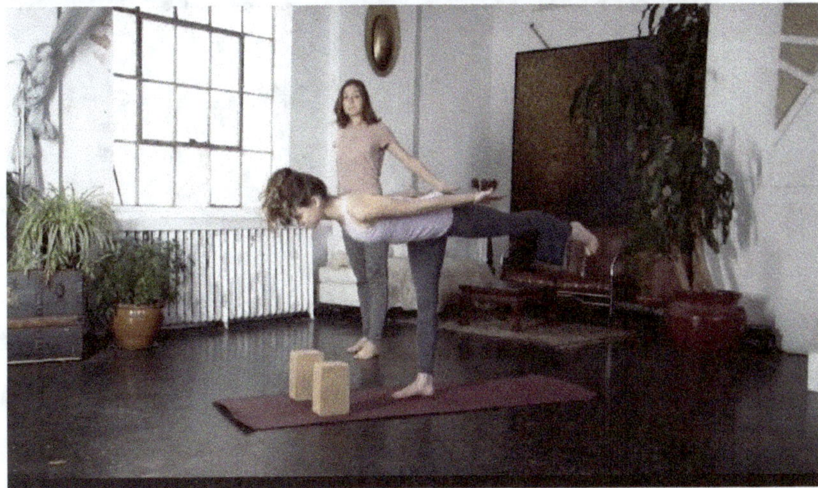

Step-by-Step Instructions:

1. Stand with your feet hip-width apart.

2. Shift your weight onto your right foot and lift your left leg behind you, keeping it straight.

3. Extend your arms forward, creating a straight line from your fingertips to your left heel.

4. For variation, extend your arms to the sides or overhead.

5. Hold for 30 seconds, then switch sides.

Tips:

Engage your core and keep your body in a straight line.

Focus on balancing and maintaining stability.

Video guide: **Warrior III with Arm Variations**

6. Shoulder Stand

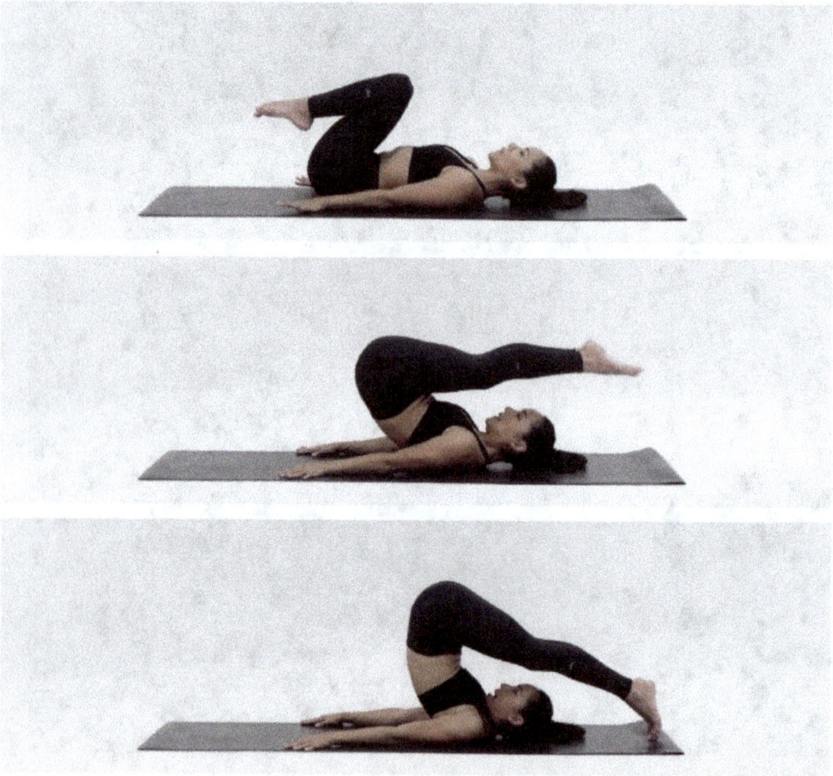

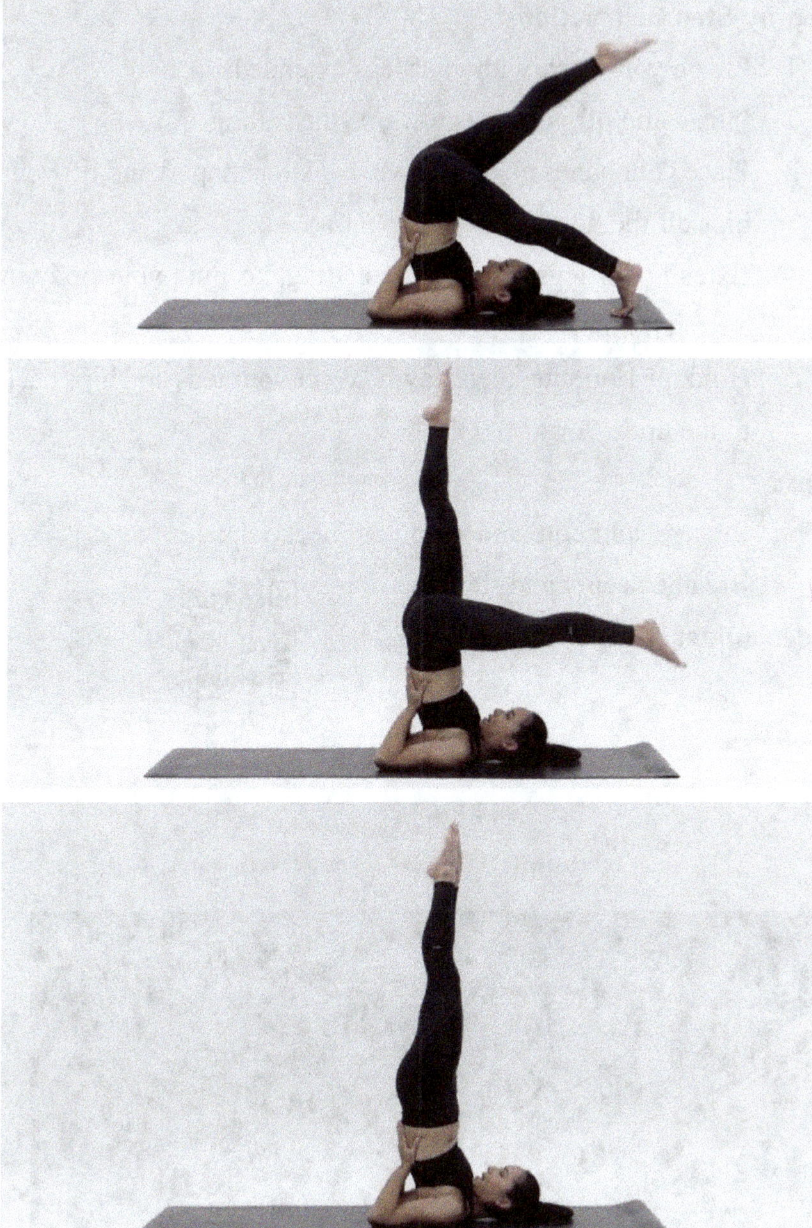

Step-by-Step Instructions:

1. Lie on your back with your legs extended.

2. Inhale and lift your legs towards the ceiling.

3. Place your hands on your lower back for support and lift your hips off the floor.

4. Extend your legs towards the ceiling, keeping your body in a straight line.

5. Hold for 1 minute, then slowly lower your legs and hips back to the floor.

Tips:

Engage your core and keep your neck relaxed.

Breathe deeply and steadily.

Video guide: Shoulder Stand Video

7. Bound Angle Pose with Forward Fold

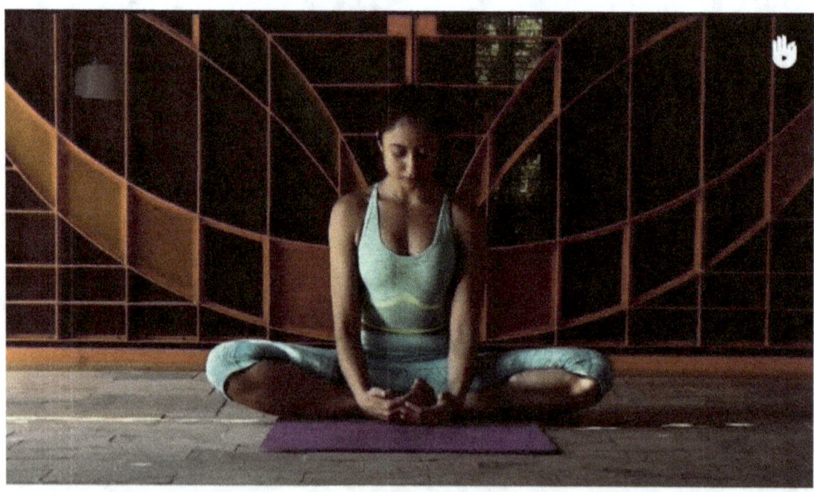

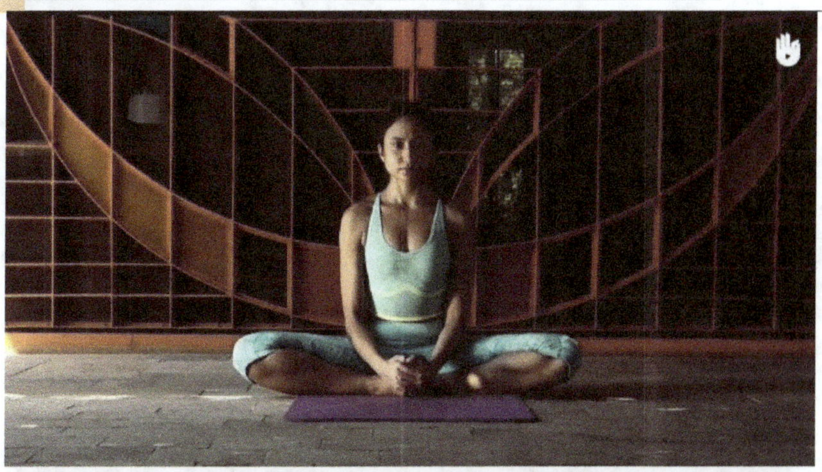

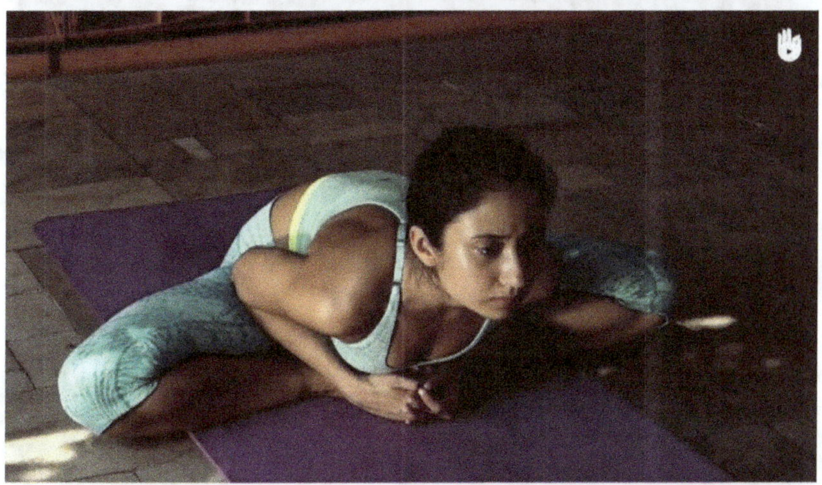

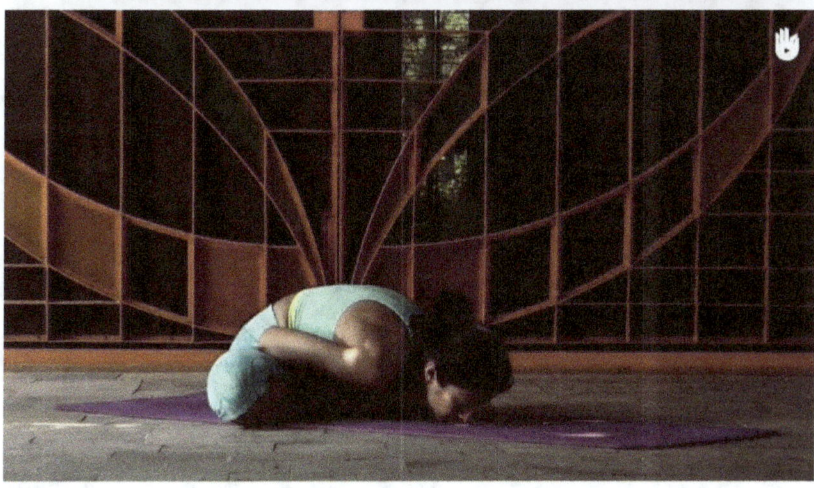

Step-by-Step Instructions:

1. Sit on the floor with your knees bent and the soles of your feet together.
2. Hold your feet with your hands and gently press your knees towards the floor.
3. Inhale, lengthen your spine, then exhale and fold forward over your feet.
4. Hold for 1-2 minutes.

Tips:

Relax your hips and allow gravity to deepen the stretch.

Use your breath to release tension.

Video guide: Bound Angle Pose Video

8. Revolved Triangle Pose

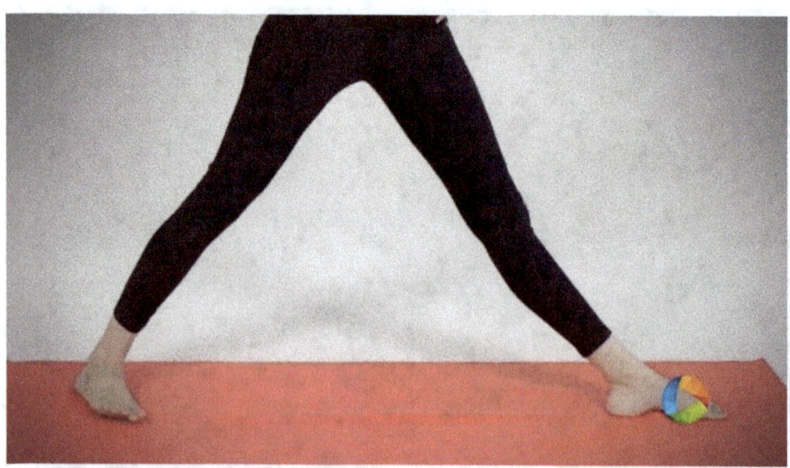

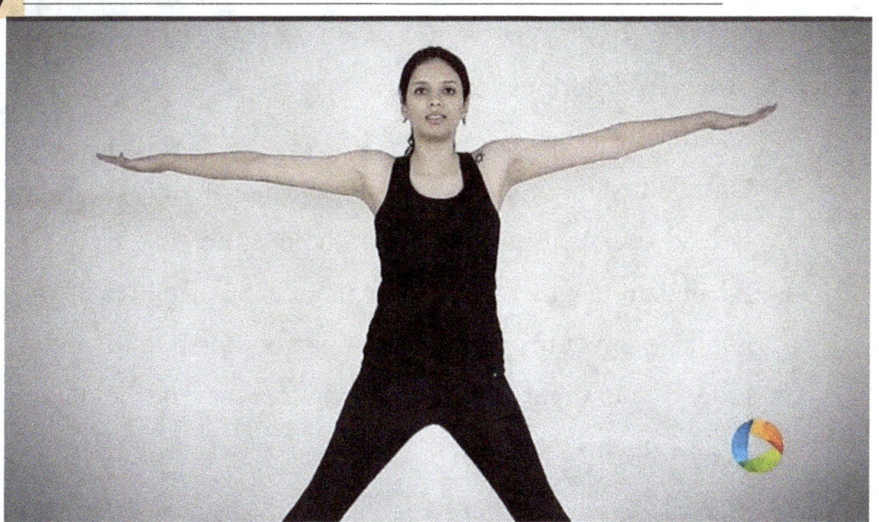

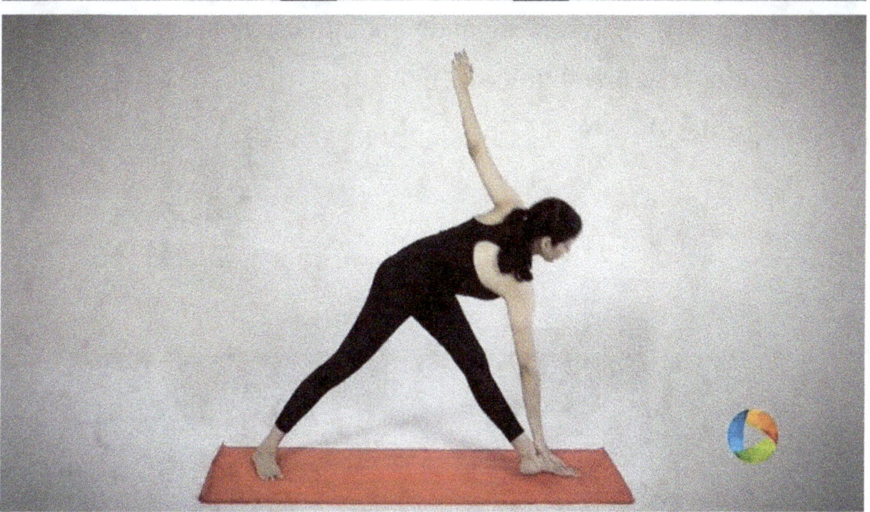

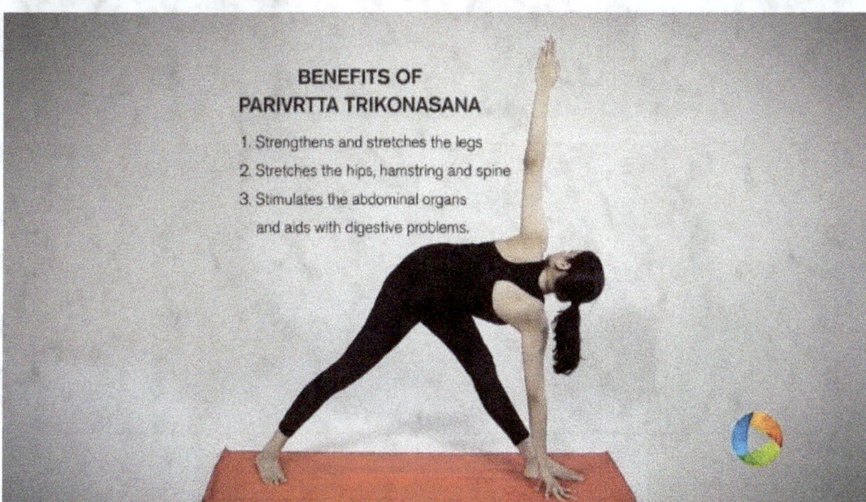
BENEFITS OF
PARIVRTTA TRIKONASANA
1. Strengthens and stretches the legs
2. Stretches the hips, hamstring and spine
3. Stimulates the abdominal organs
and aids with digestive problems.

Step-by-Step Instructions:

1. Stand with your feet wide apart.

2. Turn your right foot out and your left foot slightly in.

3. Extend your arms to the sides at shoulder height.

4. Inhale and lengthen your spine, then exhale and reach your left hand to your right foot, twisting your torso to the right.

5. Extend your right arm towards the ceiling and hold for 1 minute, then switch sides.

Tips:

Keep your spine long and your movements controlled.

Use your breath to deepen the twist.

Video guide: [Revolved Triangle Pose](#)

9. Boat Pose with Variations

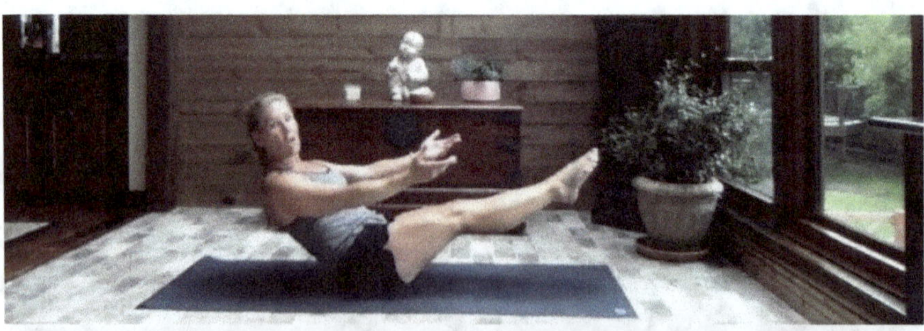

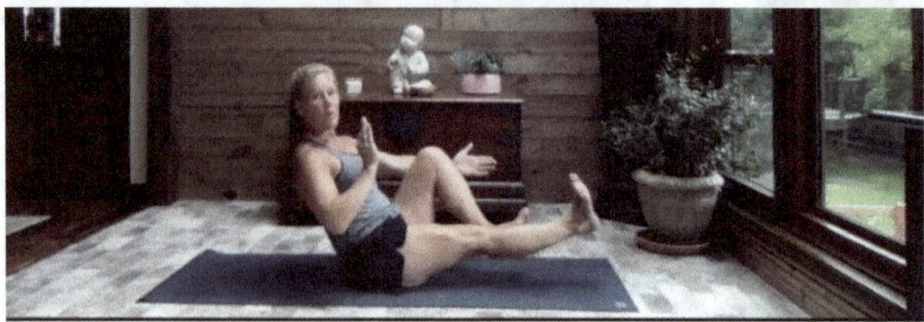

Step-by-Step Instructions:

1. Sit on the floor with your knees bent and feet flat on the floor.

2. Lean back slightly and lift your feet off the floor, balancing on your sit bones.

3. Extend your arms forward and straighten your legs to create a V shape with your body.

4. For variation, lower and lift your legs or twist your torso from side to side.

5. Hold for 30 seconds to 1 minute.

Tips:

Engage your core and keep your movements controlled.

Breathe deeply and steadily.

Video guide: Boat Pose Video Boat Pose with Variations 2

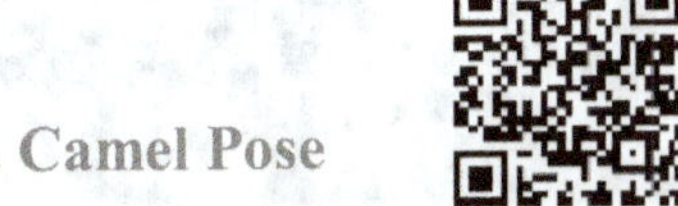

10. Camel Pose

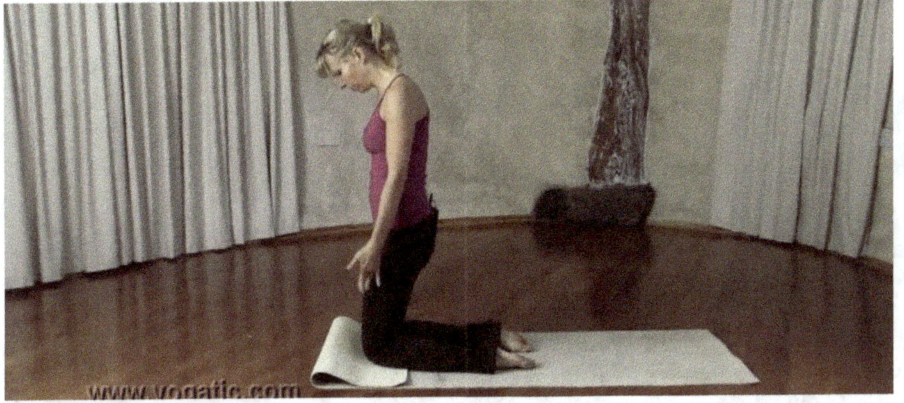

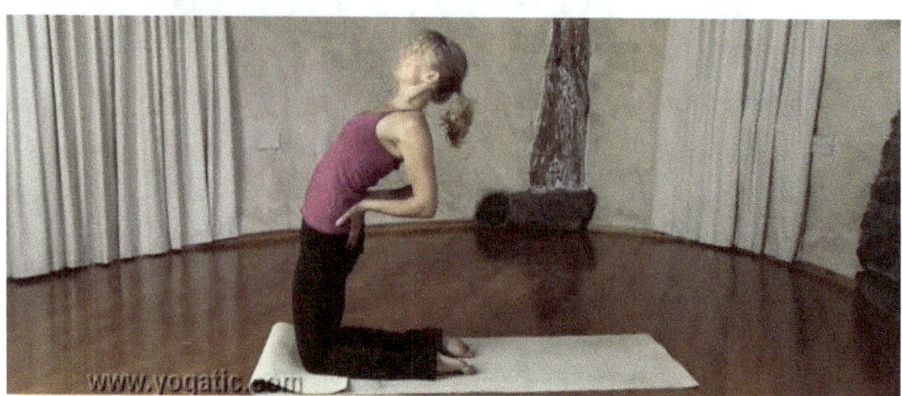

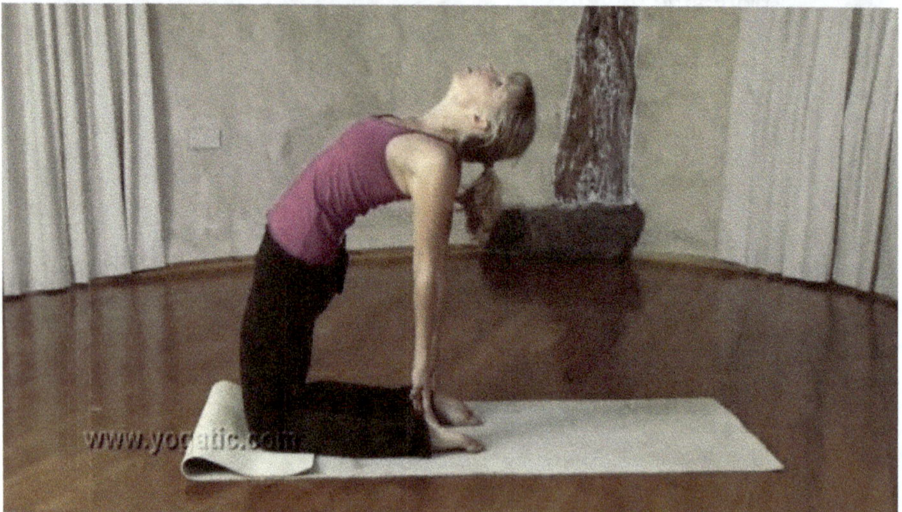

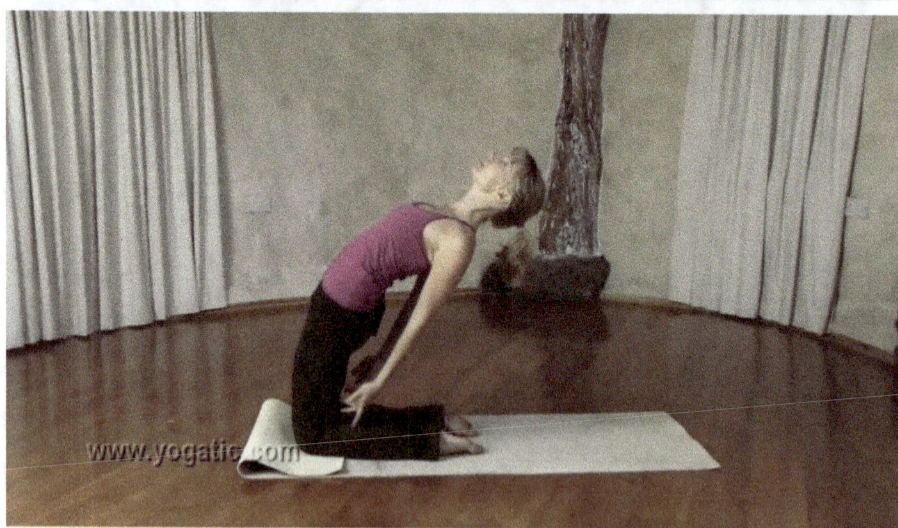

Step-by-Step Instructions:

1. Kneel on the floor with your knees hip-width apart and your hands on your lower back.

2. Inhale and lift your chest, arching your back.

3. Reach your hands back to your heels, keeping your hips over your knees.

4. Hold for 30 seconds to 1 minute, then slowly return to the starting position.

Tips:

Engage your core and keep your neck relaxed.

Breathe deeply and steadily.

Video guide: Camel Pose Video

Combining Movements for a Full-Body Practice

To create a full-body practice, combine the advanced exercises into a seamless sequence. Here's a suggested routine:

1. Warm-up: Standing Balance Series (Tree Pose and Dancer's Pose)

2. Spinal Mobility: Advanced Spinal Twist

3. Core Strength: Crow Pose and Boat Pose with Variations

4. Hip Flexibility: Pigeon Pose with Forward Fold and Bound Angle Pose with Forward Fold

5. Balance and Strength: Warrior III with Arm Variations and Revolved Triangle Pose

6. Inversion: Shoulder Stand

7. Backbend: Camel Pose

8. Cool-down: Gentle forward bends and deep breathing exercises

Role of Somatic Therapy

Understanding How Somatic Exercises Aid in Trauma Recovery

Somatic therapy focuses on the mind-body connection and how physical practices can help process and release trauma. Here's how somatic exercises play a crucial role in trauma recovery:

1. **Body Awareness:** Somatic exercises enhance body awareness, helping individuals recognize and understand the physical manifestations of trauma, such as muscle tension, pain, or restricted movement.

2. **Release of Tension:** Through gentle, mindful movements, somatic exercises help release stored tension and stress in the body, which is often a result of trauma.

3. **Regulation of the Nervous System:** Somatic exercises promote relaxation and the activation of the parasympathetic nervous system, aiding in the regulation of the nervous system and reducing symptoms of trauma, such as hypervigilance or anxiety.

4. **Emotional Processing:** By reconnecting with the body, individuals can access and process emotions associated with trauma, facilitating emotional healing and integration.

Case Studies and Professional Insights

1. **Case Study 1: Sarah's Journey to Healing**
   - **Background:** Sarah, a survivor of a traumatic car accident, experienced chronic pain and anxiety.
   - **Intervention:** Through somatic therapy, Sarah engaged in gentle movement practices, focusing on

breathing and body awareness.

- o **Outcome:** Over time, Sarah reported reduced pain, improved mobility, and a significant decrease in anxiety levels. She felt more connected to her body and more in control of her emotions.

2. **Case Study 2: John's Path to Recovery**
   - o **Background:** John, a military veteran, struggled with PTSD and chronic muscle tension.
   - o **Intervention:** John participated in somatic exercises that included deep breathing, grounding techniques, and mindful movement.
   - o **Outcome:** John experienced a reduction in PTSD symptoms, improved sleep quality, and a greater sense of calm. He found the practices empowering and integral to his recovery process.

Professional Insights:

Expert Opinion: Dr. Emily Johnson, a somatic therapist, emphasizes the importance of integrating somatic practices into trauma therapy. "Somatic exercises offer a safe and effective way to reconnect with the body and process trauma. They empower individuals to take an active role in their healing journey."

Therapeutic Value: Somatic therapy is recognized for its holistic approach, addressing both the physical and emotional aspects of trauma. It provides tools for self-regulation, resilience, and long-term recovery.

Visual Aids

Progressive Exercise Diagrams

Detailed diagrams will illustrate the advanced exercises, showing key movements and muscle engagement.

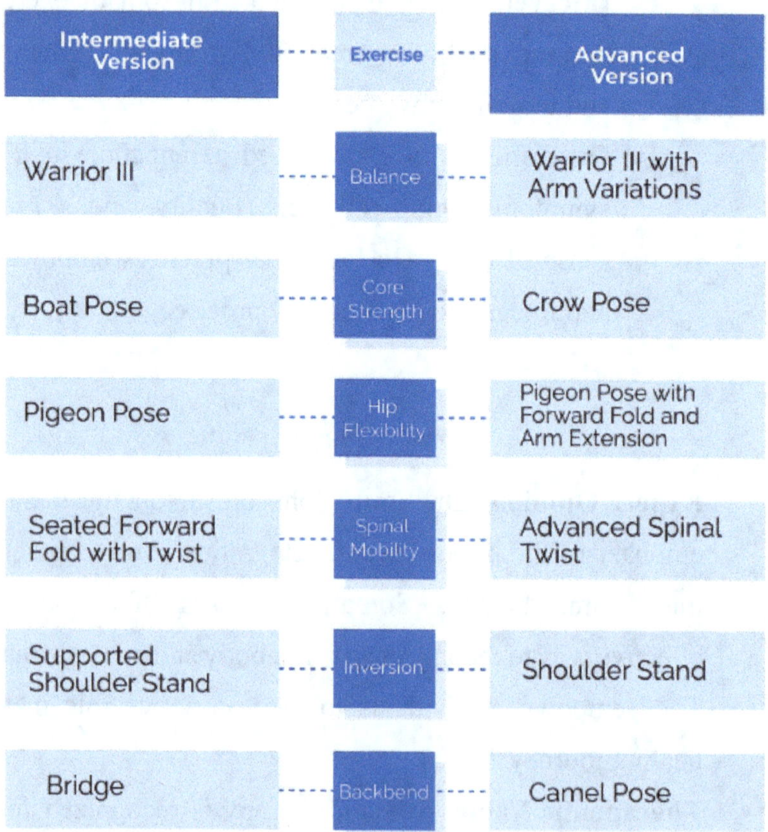

Video Links for Guided Sessions

1. **Standing Balance Series:** Standing Balance Series Video
2. **Advanced Spinal Twist:** Advanced Spinal Twist Video

3. **Crow Pose:** [Crow Pose Video](#)

4. **Pigeon Pose with Forward Fold and Arm Extension:** [Pigeon pose](#)

5. **Warrior III with Arm Variations:** [Warrior III with Arm Variations](#)

6. **Shoulder Stand:** [Shoulder Stand Video](#)

7. **Bound Angle Pose with Forward Fold:** [Bound Angle Pose Video](#)

8. **Revolved Triangle Pose:** [Revolved Triangle Pose](#)

9. **Boat Pose with Variations:** [Boat Pose Video](#) [Boat Pose with Variations 2](#)

10. **Camel Pose:** [Camel Pose Video](#)

By incorporating these advanced somatic exercises and combining them into a full-body practice, you can significantly enhance your physical and mental well-being. Understanding how somatic exercises aid in trauma recovery and exploring real-life case studies provides a deeper appreciation of the therapeutic potential of these practices.

This chapter equips you with detailed instructions, professional insights, and visual aids to help you deepen your somatic practice and integrate these advanced techniques into your daily life for sustained well-being and healing.

Chapter 7: Somatic Exercises for Specific Needs

Tailoring Exercises

Somatic exercises can be customized to meet the diverse needs of different individuals. Whether you are young or old, recovering from an injury, or managing chronic pain, these modifications ensure that you can safely and effectively benefit from somatic practices.

Modifications for Different Age Groups and Physical Conditions

1. **Children and Adolescents:**
   - **Focus:** Incorporate playful and engaging movements to maintain interest and enthusiasm.
   - **Modifications:** Use animal-themed exercises like "Cat-Cow Stretch" and "Bear Walk" to make the practice fun.
   - **Duration:** Keep sessions short (10-15 minutes) to match their attention spans.
2. **Adults:**
   - **Focus:** Address stress, posture, and flexibility issues common in adults.
   - **Modifications:** Include exercises like "Forward Bend" and "Spinal Twist" to relieve tension from

long periods of sitting.

- o **Duration:** Aim for 20-30 minutes of practice daily.

3. **Seniors:**

- o **Focus:** Enhance mobility, balance, and joint health.
- o **Modifications:** Use chair-supported versions of exercises such as "Seated Forward Fold" and "Chair Pose."
- o **Duration:** Keep sessions gentle and around 15-20 minutes, with emphasis on slow, controlled movements.

Special Considerations for Chronic Pain, Injury Recovery, and Mental Health

1. **Chronic Pain:**

- o **Focus:** Gentle movements to reduce pain and improve mobility.
- o **Modifications:** Use exercises like "Pelvic Tilt" and "Gentle Neck Rolls" to relieve tension without straining the body.
- o **Duration:** Short sessions (10-15 minutes) performed multiple times a day can be more effective.

2. **Injury Recovery:**

- o **Focus:** Gradual reintroduction of movement to avoid re-injury.
- o **Modifications:** Start with passive movements and progress to active exercises like "Supported Bridge" and "Gentle Arm Circles."
- o **Duration:** Begin with 5-10 minute sessions,

gradually increasing as recovery progresses.

3. **Mental Health:**

   o **Focus:** Incorporate exercises that promote relaxation and reduce anxiety.

   o **Modifications:** Include deep breathing exercises and meditative movements like "Body Scan Meditation" and "Reclining Bound Angle Pose."

   o **Duration:** Aim for 15-20 minutes of practice, focusing on mindfulness and breath control.

Creating Personalized Routines

Designing a personalized exercise plan involves assessing your unique needs and setting realistic goals. Here's a step-by-step guide to creating a tailored somatic routine:

1. **Assess Your Needs:**

   o **Physical Condition:** Consider any physical limitations, chronic pain, or injuries.

   o **Goals:** Determine what you hope to achieve—whether it's improving flexibility, reducing stress, or enhancing overall well-being.

   o **Preferences:** Choose exercises that you enjoy and feel comfortable performing.

2. **Set Realistic Goals:**

   o **Short-Term Goals:** Set achievable goals for the next few weeks. For example, aim to practice for 10 minutes daily.

   o **Long-Term Goals:** Think about what you want to achieve in the next few months. This could be improving posture or reducing chronic pain.

3. **Design Your Routine:**

   o **Warm-Up:** Start with gentle movements to prepare your body, such as "Shoulder Rolls" and "Ankle Circles."

   o **Main Exercises:** Choose 4-5 key exercises that address your specific needs. For example, include "Hip Opener" for flexibility and "Diaphragmatic Breathing" for relaxation.

   o **Cool-Down:** End with calming exercises to relax your body, like "Forward Bend" and "Body Scan Meditation."

4. **Adjust as Needed:**

   o **Listen to Your Body:** Modify your routine based on how you feel. If an exercise causes discomfort, adjust the movement or reduce the intensity.

   o **Track Progress:** Keep a journal to note your progress and any changes in how you feel. Adjust your routine based on your observations.

Visual Aids

Customizable Routine Templates

Here are examples of customizable routine templates for different needs:

1. **Routine Template for Adults:**

   o **Warm-Up:** Shoulder Rolls (2 minutes)

   o **Main Exercises:**

> Cat-Cow Stretch (3 minutes)
>
> Forward Bend (3 minutes)
>
> Spinal twist (3 minutes)

- o **Cool-Down:** Body Scan Meditation (2 minutes)
- o **Total Duration:** 10 minutes

2. **Routine Template for Seniors:**
   - o **Warm-Up:** Ankle Circles (2 minutes)
   - o **Main Exercises:**

     > Seated Forward Fold (3 minutes)
     >
     > Gentle Neck Rolls (3 minutes)
     >
     > Chair Pose (3 minutes)

   - o **Cool-Down:** Diaphragmatic Breathing (2 minutes)
   - o **Total Duration:** 10 minutes

Modified Exercises

To help visualize the exercises, here are illustrations of modified versions of common somatic exercises:

1. **Chair-Supported Forward Bend:** This shows a person sitting in a chair, bending forward with hands reaching towards the feet.

2. **Seated Cat-Cow Stretch:** Depicts a person sitting on a chair, performing the cat-cow stretch with back arching and rounding.

3. **Gentle Neck Rolls:** Illustrates a person sitting comfortably, rolling their neck in a circular motion.

4. **Supported Bridge Pose:** Shows a person lying on their back with a yoga block or cushion under their lower back for support.

These visual aids and templates will assist you in creating a personalized somatic routine that suits your specific needs and goals. By tailoring exercises and incorporating them into your daily life, you can achieve greater body awareness, reduce discomfort, and enhance overall well-being.

Somatic Exercise
Comprehensive Mind-Body Practices for Holistic Health and Wellness

These visual aids and templates will assist you in creating a personalized somatic routine that suits your specific needs and goals. By tailoring exercises and incorporating them into your daily life, you can achieve greater body awareness, reduce discomfort, and enhance overall well-being.

Chapter 8: Resources and Further Learning

Continuing Your Journey

The journey to body awareness and healing through somatic exercises is an ongoing process. Here are some resources to help you continue learning and deepening your practice.

Recommended Books, Websites, and Professionals for Further Learning

Books:

1. **"The Body Keeps the Score" by Bessel van der Kolk**
2. **"The Feldenkrais Method: Teaching by Handling" by Yochanan Rywerant**
   - A guide to the Feldenkrais Method, focusing on using touch to teach body awareness.

Websites:

1. **Somatic Experiencing® Trauma Institute**
   - Provides information on somatic experiencing, a body-focused therapy for trauma.
2. **The Feldenkrais Guild of North America**
   - Offers resources on the Feldenkrais Method, including practitioner directories and learning materials.
3. **International Association for Dance Medicine & Science (IADMS)**
   - Provides resources on somatic practices in dance and movement education.

Professionals:

1. **Dr. Peter Levine**
   - A pioneer in somatic experiencing, offering workshops and training programs.

2. **Moshe Feldenkrais Practitioners**
   - Certified practitioners who teach the Feldenkrais Method.
   - Find a practitioner

How to Stay Updated on New Developments in Somatic Practices

1. **Subscribe to Newsletters:**
   - Many organizations and professionals offer newsletters with updates on somatic practices, research, and events.
   - Example: Somatic Experiencing® Trauma Institute Newsletter

2. **Follow Blogs and Online Journals:**
   - Blogs and journals often publish articles on the latest developments in somatic practices.
   - Example: The Feldenkrais Method Blog

3. **Attend Workshops and Conferences:**
   - Participating in workshops and conferences provides opportunities to learn from experts and stay informed about new techniques.
   - Example: IADMS Annual Conference

Community and Support

Building a supportive community is crucial for sustaining your somatic practice. Here are ways to connect with others:

Joining Groups, Forums, and Classes for Ongoing Support

1. **Online Forums and Groups:**
   - **Facebook Groups:** Search for groups dedicated to somatic practices, such as "Somatic Healing" or "Feldenkrais Practitioners and Enthusiasts."
2. **Local Classes and Workshops:**
   - Check local wellness centres, yoga studios, and community centers for classes and workshops on somatic practices.
   - Example: Search for "somatic yoga classes near me" on Google.
3. **Professional Associations:**
   - Joining professional associations can provide access to resources, networking opportunities, and continuing education.
   - Example: **American Dance Therapy Association**

Sharing Your Progress and Experiences with Others

1. **Start a Journal or Blog:**
   - Document your journey and share insights, challenges, and successes with others.
   - Platforms like WordPress or Medium can help you reach a wider audience.
2. **Social Media:**
   - Share your progress and connect with like-minded individuals on platforms like Instagram, Twitter, and Facebook.
   - Use hashtags like #somatichealing, #bodyawareness, and #mindfulmovement.

3. **Participate in Online Challenges:**
   - Join or create challenges that encourage regular practice and community support.
   - Example: Host a 30-day somatic exercise challenge on Instagram and invite others to join.

Lists of Resources with Brief Descriptions

1. **Books:**
   - "The Body Keeps the Score" by Bessel van der Kolk Explores the impact of trauma on the body and mind.
   - "Somatics" by Thomas Hanna: Introduction to somatic practices for health and flexibility.
   - "The Feldenkrais Method" by Yochanan Rywerant: Guide to teaching body awareness through touch.

2. **Websites:**
   - Somatic Experiencing® Trauma Institute: Information and resources on somatic experiencing.
   - The Feldenkrais Guild of North America: Resources and practitioner directories for the Feldenkrais Method.
   - International Association for Dance Medicine & Science (IADMS): Resources on somatic practices in dance and movement education.

3. **Professionals:**
   - Dr. Peter Levine: Workshops and training in somatic experiencing.
   - Moshe Feldenkrais Practitioners: Certified practitioners teaching the Feldenkrais Method.

Online Communities and Support Networks

1. **Somatic Experiencing® Trauma Institute Newsletter:** Subscribe

2. **Feldenkrais Method Blog:** Blog

3. **American Dance Therapy Association:** ADTA

4. **IADMS Annual Conference:** Conference

These resources, communities, and support networks will help you continue your journey into somatic practices, providing ongoing learning, support, and inspiration. By staying connected and informed, you can deepen your practice and enhance your overall well-being.

Checklists for Building a Somatic Routine

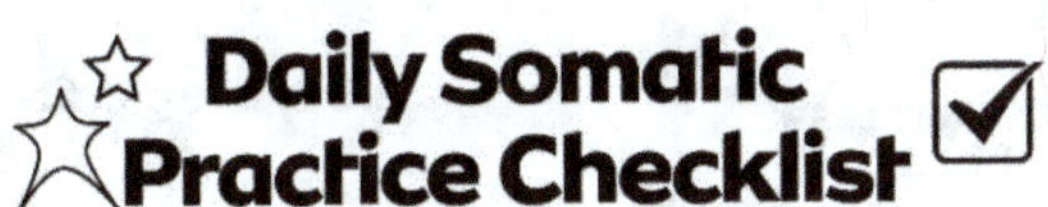

Daily Somatic Practice Checklist

1. Set a specific time for practice

Morning ☐
Afternoon ☐
Evening ☐

2. Create a dedicated practice space

Quiet area ☐
Comfortable mat ☐
Minimal distractions ☐

3. Start with a few minutes of practice

5 minutes ☐
10 minutes ☐
15 minutes ☐

4. Use reminders and cues

Phone alarm ☐
Sticky notes ☐
Visual cues ☐

5. Integrate exercises with daily activities

Morning stretch ☐
Lunchtime break ☐
Evening relaxation ☐

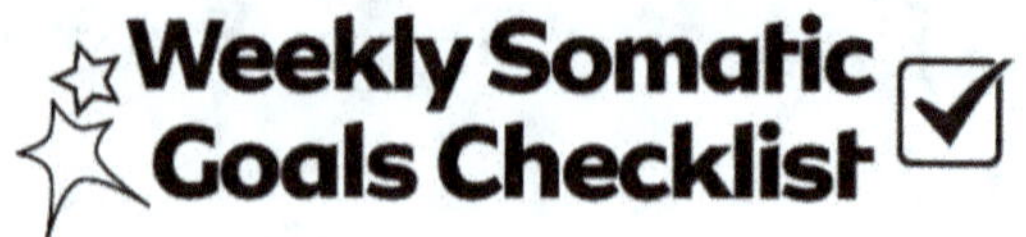

Weekly Somatic Goals Checklist

1. Practice somatic exercises at least 5 times a week

Monday ☐

Tuesday ☐

Wednesday ☐

Thursday ☐

Friday ☐

Saturday ☐

Sunday ☐

2. Increase practice duration gradually

10 minutes ☐

20 minutes ☐

30 minutes ☐

3. Incorporate a variety of exercises

Breathing exercises ☐

Centering techniques ☐

Movement sequences ☐

4. Reflect on progress and adjust routine as needed

Journal entries ☐

Self-assessment ☐

Feedback from others ☐

5. Join a somatic exercise class or online community for support

Local class ☐

Online group ☐

Social media community ☐

Additional Pictures of Somatic Poses

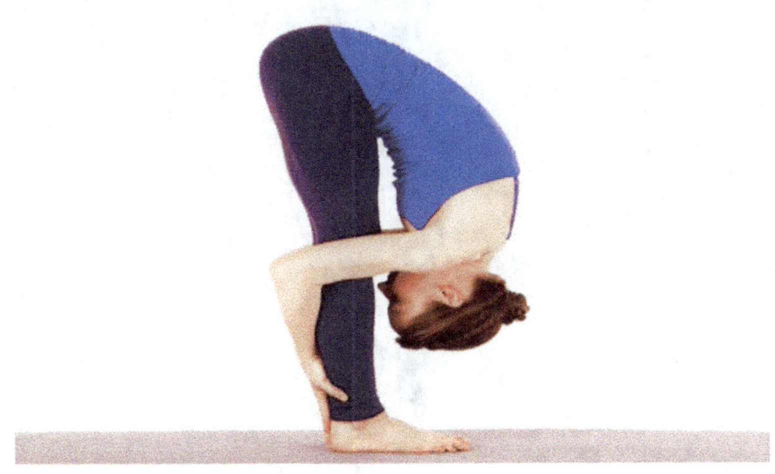

The forward bend

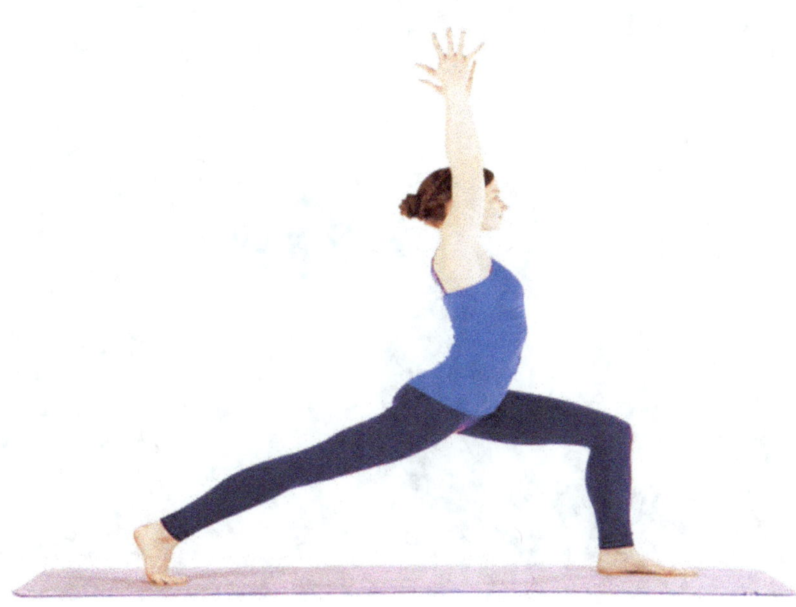

High Lunge: Left

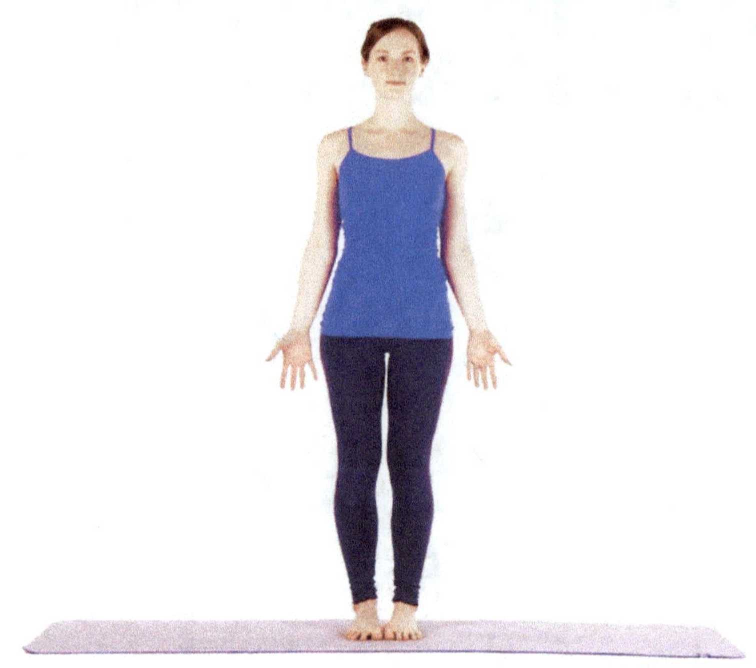

Mountain

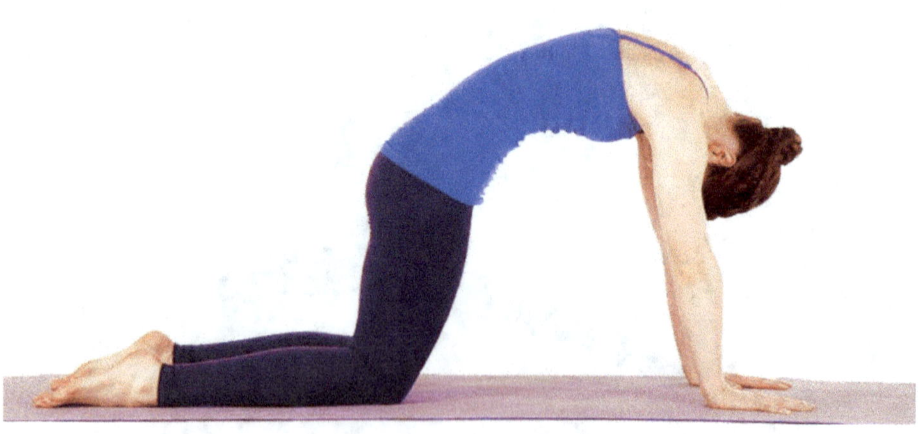

The Cat Pose

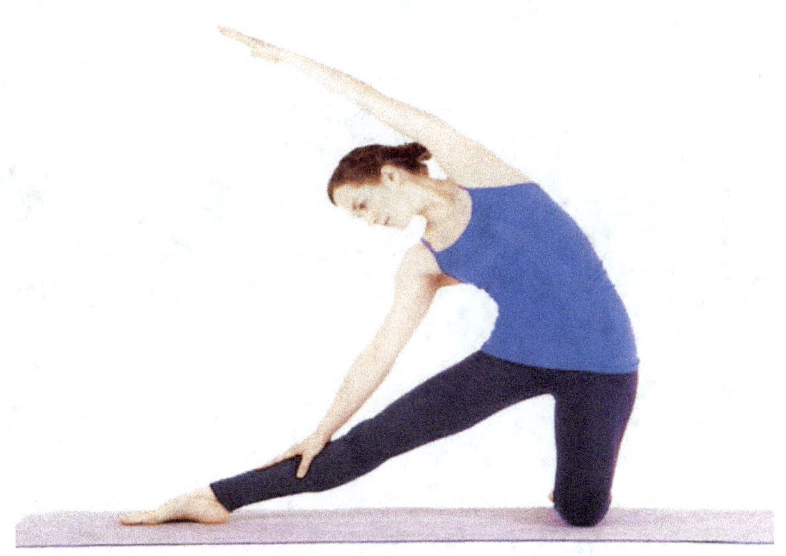

Gate: Right

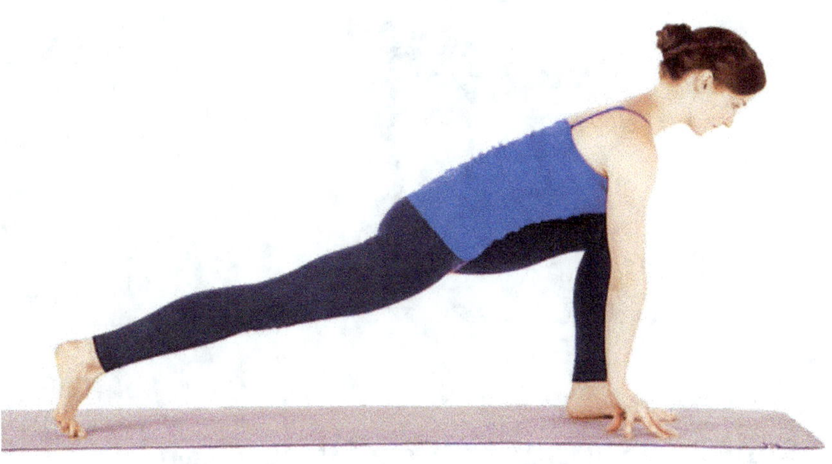

Runner's Lunge: Left

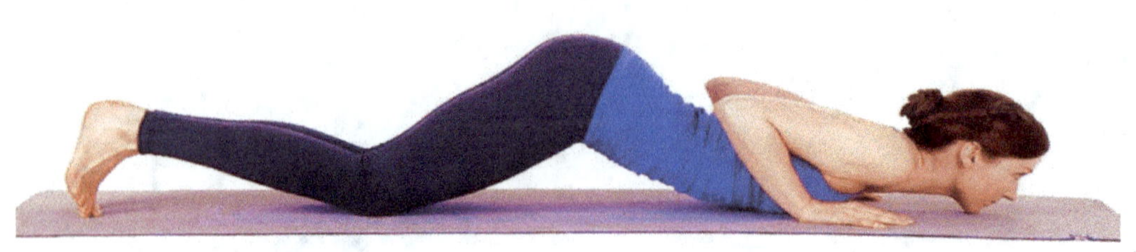

Chest Chin

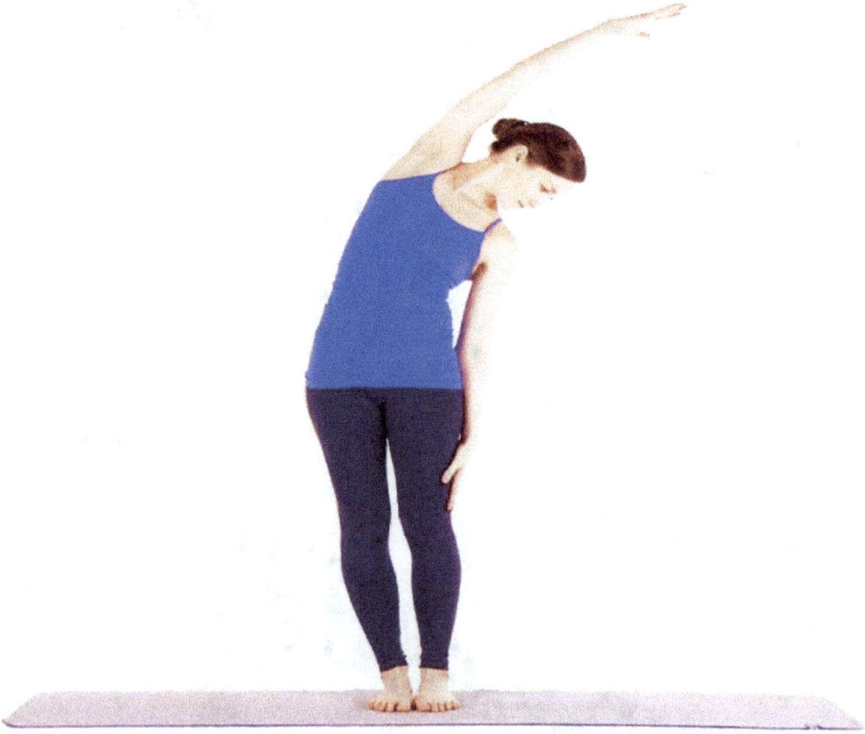

Standing Supported Side Stretch: Left

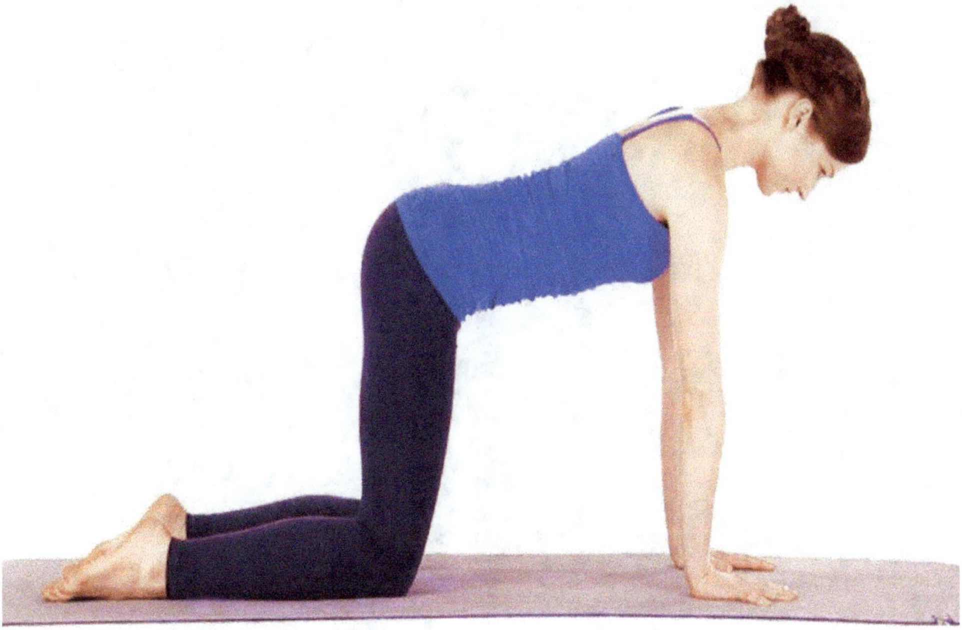

Table Top

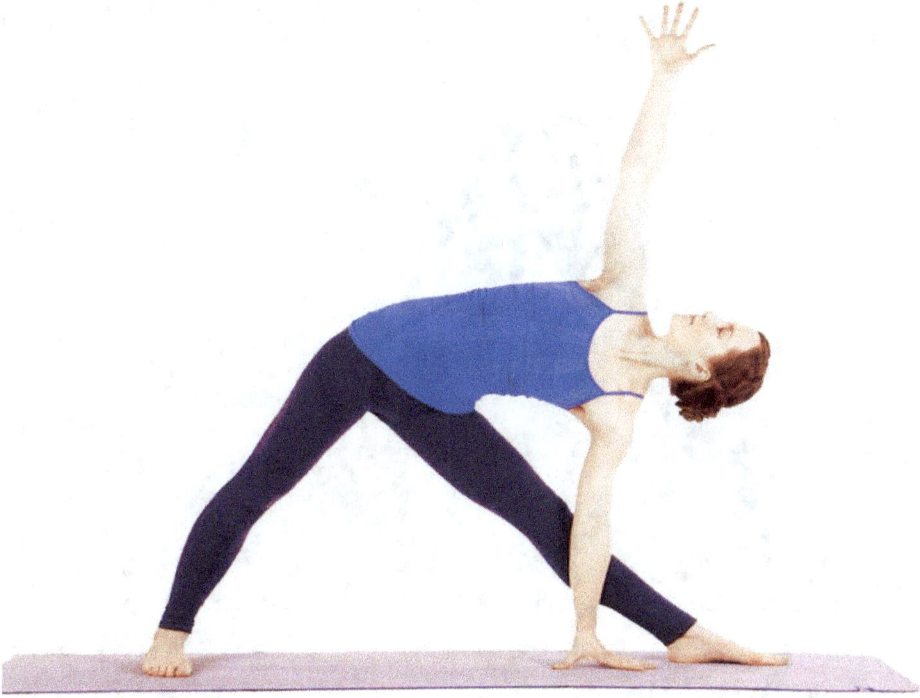

Triangle: Left

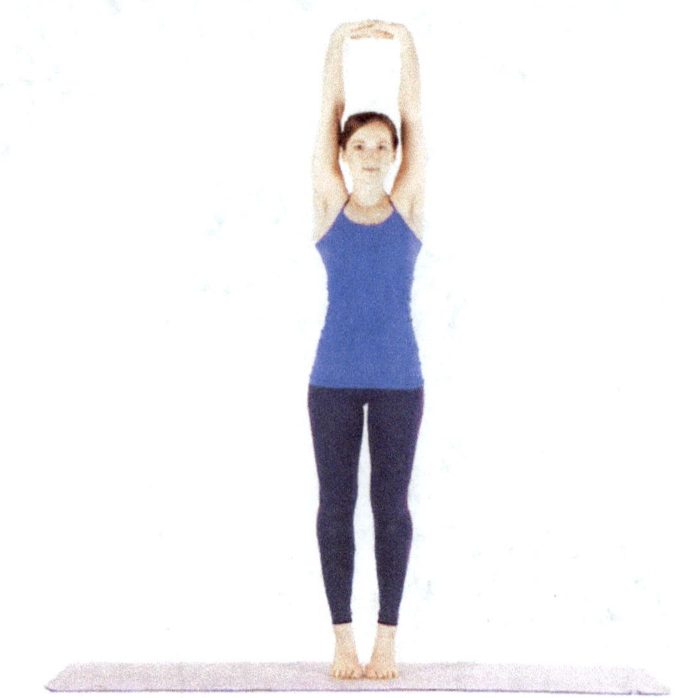

Palm Tree

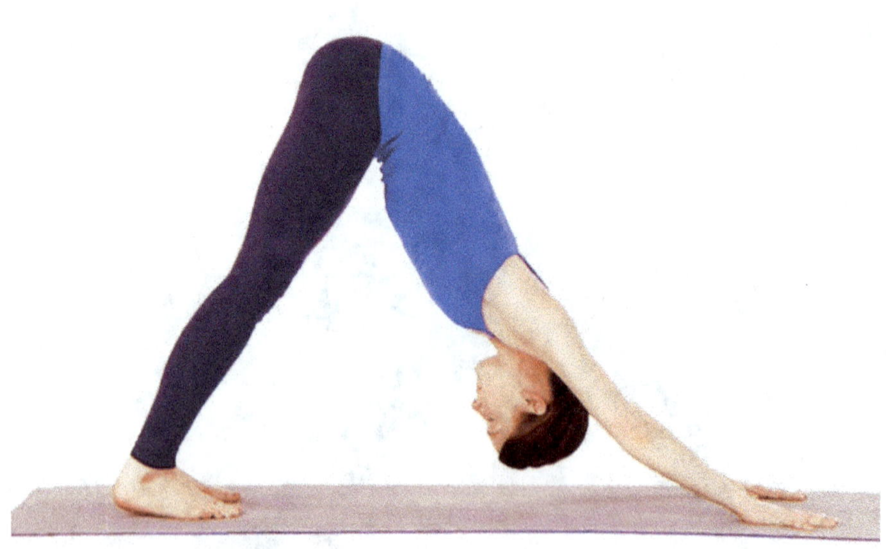

Downward Dog

www.ingramcontent.com/pod-product-compliance
Lightning Source LLC
Chambersburg PA
CBHW071041250726
48653CB00005B/1941